MANAGING POST-OBTURATION PAIN AND SWELLING IN NON-SURGICAL ENDODONTICS

Kingsley Oluyomi Obanubi

TABLE OF CONTENTS

PREFACE

Pain and swelling that occur after root canal treatment have long challenged both clinicians and researchers. These postoperative symptoms often appear in the quiet hours after a patient leaves the dental chair, raising questions about technique, biology, and the delicate balance between mechanical intervention and tissue response. Although endodontic therapy continues to advance through improved instruments, materials, and technology, the problem of post obturation discomfort remains one of the most significant indicators of treatment quality and patient satisfaction. Understanding why these symptoms occur and how they can be prevented or managed has become an essential part of contemporary endodontic practice.

This book was developed to address that need through a research based and clinically informed approach. It brings together current scientific literature, clinical experience, and evidence generated from multiple endodontic studies, including peer reviewed publications authored by the same researcher whose work forms the foundation of this text. The goal is to provide clarity on both the mechanisms and management of post obturation complications in a way that supports clinicians who strive to deliver predictable and comfortable outcomes for their patients.

At the core of this work is the belief that a successful root canal treatment is defined not only by radiographic healing or technical precision, but also by the patient's postoperative experience. Pain and swelling can affect trust, influence long term perceptions of dental care, and complicate treatment plans. For that reason, this book examines the biological and mechanical contributors to postoperative symptoms with a depth that reflects their clinical importance. Readers will find discussions on inflammatory pathways, microbial survival, instrument related trauma, obturation quality, patient specific factors, and other variables that influence postoperative responses.

Equally important is the emphasis on prevention. Evidence based strategies for reducing postoperative discomfort shape a significant portion of this work. These strategies include advances in irrigation systems, safer instrumentation methods, antimicrobial protocols, obturation techniques, and modern approaches to intracanal medication. By integrating current research with practical protocols, the book aims to strengthen clinical decision making and reduce the frequency of postoperative complications.

Management principles are also presented in a structured and accessible format. Clinicians often encounter situations in which postoperative pain exceeds expected limits or fails to resolve in a typical timeframe. Differentiating between normal healing patterns and pathological presentations requires skill, diagnostic discipline, and awareness of current therapeutic options. This book offers a clear guide for evaluating such cases and selecting appropriate pharmacologic and non-pharmacologic interventions.

For cases that require more than conservative care, the text explores retreatment considerations and long term clinical outcomes. These chapters support practitioners who must decide when and how to intervene without compromising the stability of surrounding tissues or the prognosis of the tooth.

This work was written with the hope that it becomes a dependable reference for clinicians, researchers, postgraduate students, and educators. The content reflects collective knowledge built over years of academic study, clinical involvement, and a commitment to improving patient comfort following endodontic procedures. It invites readers to appreciate the complexities of post obturation physiology while offering practical tools for effective prevention and management.

I am grateful to mentors, colleagues, and the broader dental community whose contributions to endodontic science continue to inspire inquiry and innovation. Their efforts make books like this possible and advance the quality of care delivered worldwide.

Ultimately, the purpose of this book is to support better patient outcomes. When postoperative pain is minimized and swelling is properly controlled, patients experience greater confidence in their treatment, and clinicians achieve results that reflect the highest standards of modern endodontics. It is my hope that the knowledge shared in these pages contributes meaningfully to that goal.

FOREWORD

The practice of endodontics has reached a stage where scientific understanding, clinical experience, and technological advancement intersect more closely than ever before. The modern clinician has access to tools and imaging systems that previous generations could only imagine, yet one persistent reality continues to challenge even the most skilled practitioners. That reality is the occurrence of post obturation pain and swelling. These complications, familiar to every endodontist and general practitioner who performs root canal therapy, remain a significant source of patient concern and professional responsibility. Even when treatment has been carried out with absolute precision, postoperative symptoms can arise unexpectedly and influence patient comfort, treatment perception, and overall clinical outcomes.

The need for a comprehensive and research grounded understanding of post obturation complications has never been greater. Endodontic therapy is increasingly shaped by patient centered care, evidence based protocols, and a demand for predictable results. As a result, clinicians are expected to understand not only how to perform a technically successful procedure but also how to anticipate, prevent, diagnose, and manage postoperative symptoms with confidence and accuracy. The gap between clinical technique and biological response has become an important area of academic inquiry, and this book stands as a timely contribution to that evolving conversation.

The author brings together an impressive body of research and clinical observation to explore the complexities surrounding post obturation pain and swelling. These chapters are grounded in scientific literature, yet they remain fully accessible to practitioners who want clear and practical explanations. Within these pages, readers will encounter detailed insights into microbial survival, inflammatory mediators, neural mechanisms, mechanical irritation, and patient specific variables that influence postoperative outcomes. The material is presented in a manner that strengthens the clinician's ability to interpret symptoms based on biological reasoning rather than assumption or routine.

One of the strengths of this book is its commitment to integrative understanding. Many texts in endodontics address instrumentation, irrigation, and obturation techniques as isolated steps. This book presents them as interconnected processes that collectively influence the likelihood of postoperative complications. By discussing how apical extrusion, incomplete microbial control, obturation pressure, canal anatomy, and procedural variables converge, the author provides a framework that mirrors real clinical conditions. This holistic approach allows clinicians to refine every stage of treatment with the goal of minimizing postoperative inflammation.

Prevention is presented not as a theoretical ideal but as a tangible, achievable outcome. Readers will find guidance on contemporary irrigation strategies, improved debridement efficiency, antimicrobial protocols, canal preparation techniques, and obturation methods that have demonstrated success in reducing postoperative discomfort. These sections draw from both classical research and recent advancements in endodontic science. The emphasis on prevention encourages clinicians to approach each case with foresight and planning, understanding that postoperative pain is not merely a reaction to obturation but often a consequence of earlier procedural factors.

Equally important is the attention given to clinical assessment and diagnostic clarity. Post obturation symptoms often create uncertainty for both patients and clinicians. Distinguishing between expected healing responses and complications that require intervention demands skill and a thorough understanding of endodontic pathology. This book offers structured diagnostic guidance, including the use of pain scales, radiographic interpretation, percussion and palpation responses, and symptom progression patterns. By articulating clear criteria for evaluation, the author equips clinicians to make informed and timely decisions.

The chapters devoted to management strategies are especially valuable for practitioners in everyday clinical environments. Pain that persists beyond expected limits, swelling that suggests microbial activity, and flare ups that disrupt treatment plans are situations that every clinician encounters. The book presents pharmacologic protocols, patient communication strategies, and stepwise treatment approaches that support predictable symptom resolution. These discussions are informed by current research and align with contemporary standards of care.

Furthermore, the inclusion of content related to retreatment decisions and long term prognostic considerations enriches the book's practical application. There are moments in clinical practice when earlier interventions require reassessment, and the guidance offered here helps clinicians navigate those decisions with accuracy and ethical clarity. Retreatment is never a simple step, and the author emphasizes the importance of understanding both the mechanical and biological factors that influence the success of such procedures.

Beyond its academic strength, this book carries a deeper message about the philosophy of care. Endodontic treatment is not limited to technical execution. It is a biological interaction that affects patient comfort, trust, and long term oral health. By examining postoperative symptoms through a scientific and compassionate lens, the book reflects a dedication to improving both clinical outcomes and patient experiences. It encourages clinicians to recognize that managing postoperative pain is not merely a professional obligation. It is an essential part of the therapeutic journey and a reflection of the clinician's commitment to excellence.

The scientific community continues to benefit from works that connect evidence with clinical decision making. This book stands among such contributions. Its clarity, structure, and depth make it suitable for postgraduate students, practicing clinicians, researchers, and educators who seek a deeper understanding of postoperative complications in non surgical endodontics. It supports both academic exploration and practical application, offering readers the tools they need to refine their practice and raise the standard of patient care.

It is with great respect for the author's dedication to research, clinical insight, and scholarly advancement that I present this foreword. May this work serve as a useful companion for clinicians at all stages of their professional journey and contribute meaningfully to the ongoing effort to provide safe, effective, and comfortable endodontic treatment for all patients.

INTRODUCTION

Root canal therapy remains one of the most widely performed procedures in restorative dentistry, and its success depends on a sophisticated interplay of biology, technique, and clinical judgment. Although significant progress has been made in instrument design, imaging systems, irrigation technologies, and obturation materials, postoperative pain and swelling continue to represent some of the most common complications encountered after treatment. These symptoms, while often transient, can influence a patient's perception of care, alter compliance with follow up instructions, and create uncertainty for both clinician and patient. Understanding their cause, prevention, and management is therefore an essential part of modern endodontic practice.

This book was developed to address those issues with an approach that brings scientific knowledge, clinical evidence, and practical experience together in a unified and accessible format. The intention is not only to describe postoperative complications but to explain them in a way that strengthens clinical reasoning and guides decision making. Endodontic treatment occurs within a biological environment that responds to every step of the procedure. The shaping of canals, the removal of microbial biofilms, the irrigation dynamics, and the quality of the obturation collectively determine how periapical tissues will react once treatment is completed. When these processes interact with patient specific factors, they can produce postoperative symptoms that range from mild discomfort to significant swelling or flare ups.

Understanding the etiology of these reactions begins with a study of the biological and mechanical factors that influence periapical tissues. Microbial persistence remains one of the primary contributors to postoperative pain, and even small numbers of residual microorganisms can trigger an inflammatory response. Mechanical irritation such as apical extrusion of debris or over instrumentation can also provoke tissue responses that manifest as pain or swelling. In addition, the materials used during obturation, the thermal effect of certain techniques, and the physical properties of sealers may interact with tissues in ways that influence postoperative outcomes. This book examines these contributors with a depth that allows clinicians to appreciate how each step of treatment influences the next.

Prevention is a central theme throughout this text. While complete elimination of postoperative symptoms is not always possible, many techniques and strategies significantly reduce their incidence. Research supported protocols for effective irrigation, improved microbial control, and careful canal preparation are explored in detail. The goal is to provide clinicians with methods that support predictable healing by reducing the stimuli that provoke inflammatory responses. Prevention also includes attention to procedural accuracy, instrument choice, irrigation dynamics, and obturation technique. When these factors are understood as an integrated system, clinicians can reduce the likelihood of complications before the patient even leaves the operatory.

For cases in which symptoms do occur, accurate clinical assessment becomes essential. Distinguishing between expected postoperative discomfort and signs of pathology requires a clear understanding of endodontic diagnosis and the factors that influence healing. This book offers a structured approach to case evaluation, guiding clinicians through symptom characterization, radiographic interpretation, percussion and palpation findings, and functional assessment. This diagnostic clarity supports timely decision making and helps avoid unnecessary interventions.

Management of postoperative pain and swelling requires both pharmacologic and non-pharmacologic approaches. Analgesics, non-steroidal anti inflammatory medications, corticosteroids, and antibiotics all play roles under specific indications supported by evidence. Understanding when each medication is appropriate and how it should be combined with clinical care is essential for predictable relief. These topics are explored with an emphasis on safety, effectiveness, and alignment with current guidelines.

In situations where symptoms persist or worsen, deeper clinical intervention may be required. Persistent complications can arise due to microbial survival, procedural errors, unrecognized anatomical complexity, or other factors. The text describes a range of evidence based protocols for addressing these situations, including when to monitor, when to initiate retreatment, and when referral to a specialist is appropriate. By presenting a clear decision making pathway, the book supports clinicians in managing complex postoperative cases with confidence.

Finally, this work includes discussions about long term outcomes, retreatment considerations, patient communication, and the integration of new scientific findings into daily practice. Endodontics is a rapidly evolving field, and practitioners must adapt to new evidence as it emerges. This book aims to serve as both a reference and a guide for continuous learning.

The content throughout this text reflects a commitment to improving patient outcomes by advancing the understanding of postoperative physiology and strengthening clinical protocols. It is intended for clinicians, postgraduate students, educators, and researchers who seek a deeper and more structured understanding of how post obturation pain and swelling develop and how they can be effectively prevented or managed.

Above all, the goal is to support the delivery of care that is both scientifically grounded and compassionate. When clinicians understand the biological mechanisms behind postoperative symptoms and apply evidence based strategies to their work, patients benefit through improved comfort, confidence, and long term oral health. It is my hope that this book contributes meaningfully to that effort and inspires continued excellence in the practice of non-surgical endodontics.

CHAPTER 1

Understanding Post Obturation Pain and Swelling

Post obturation pain and swelling remain some of the most frequently reported postoperative complications in non-surgical endodontics. They occur even in cases where the clinician has followed accepted treatment protocols and executed the procedure with precision. For many patients, root canal therapy is associated with fear of discomfort, and postoperative pain reinforces this perception. It can influence how patients evaluate the success of treatment, how they comply with follow up care, and whether they remain confident in the clinician's ability. For practitioners, postoperative symptoms create clinical challenges that require careful assessment, communication, and appropriate management. To understand why these symptoms arise, it is necessary to examine both the biological and procedural factors that shape the patient's response after obturation.

Post obturation pain can be defined as any discomfort that develops after the final filling of the root canal system. This discomfort can range from mild tenderness during biting to spontaneous pain that interferes with daily activities. Swelling, although less common, is generally associated with inflammatory reactions or microbial activity within or around the periapical tissues. Understanding these symptoms requires a recognition that root canal therapy is an intervention within a living biological system. Even when the canal has been properly cleaned, shaped, disinfected, and sealed, the surrounding tissues continue to respond to mechanical and chemical stimuli introduced during treatment.

One of the most important considerations when examining postoperative symptoms is the role of the periapical tissues. These tissues are highly vascular and contain a variety of cells that participate in immune responses. When instrumentation, irrigation, or obturation techniques extend beyond the anatomical boundaries of the canal or when microbial remnants remain within the system, the periapical tissues react. The nature of this reaction depends on the degree of irritation and the ability of the host to modulate inflammation. Mild irritation may result in temporary discomfort that resolves within a few days. More significant irritation may lead to swelling, throbbing pain, or development of a postoperative flare up.

The causes of post obturation pain are multifactorial. Although microbial factors often receive the most attention, mechanical trauma introduced during the procedure also plays a significant role. Instrumentation can extrude dentinal debris into the periapical space, which triggers an inflammatory response. The use of irrigants can introduce chemical irritation when solutions inadvertently pass beyond the apex or when tissue reactions occur due to concentration or exposure time. The obturation process can also introduce pressure within the canal system, and materials that exit the apex can cause foreign body reactions. The combination of these factors creates conditions that stimulate nociceptors and produce pain.

Microbial persistence is one of the primary reasons postoperative symptoms occur. Even with advanced irrigation systems and antimicrobial solutions, complete elimination of microorganisms from complex canal anatomy remains challenging. Lateral canals, apical deltas, and fins can harbor bacteria that survive instrumentation. These microorganisms release toxins and metabolic products that diffuse into the periapical tissues and stimulate inflammatory responses. The host immune system reacts by recruiting inflammatory cells, increasing vascular permeability, and releasing mediators that cause pain and swelling. Understanding this biological pathway helps clinicians appreciate why postoperative symptoms sometimes occur even when the canal appears radiographically clean.

Patient related factors also influence postoperative outcomes. Each individual has a unique pain threshold, immune response, and healing capacity. Medical history, systemic conditions, and psychological state can affect how postoperative symptoms are perceived and reported. For instance, patients with heightened anxiety may interpret mild discomfort as severe pain. Individuals with diabetes or compromised immune function may experience prolonged inflammation. These variations highlight the importance of individualized patient care and effective communication.

Another essential concept in understanding postoperative pain is the difference between expected postoperative discomfort and pathological symptoms. Some degree of sensitivity is common after root canal therapy due to tissue manipulation. This discomfort usually diminishes within a few days and does not require intervention beyond standard analgesics. Pathological pain, however, presents differently. It may be persistent, intensifying, or accompanied by swelling, fever, difficulty in chewing, or systemic involvement. Recognizing these differences is crucial for making appropriate clinical decisions.

Swelling after obturation is typically associated with inflammation or microbial activity. When bacteria remain within the canal or when toxins escape into the periapical tissues, the immune response becomes more pronounced. Fluid accumulates as part of the inflammatory process, and swelling becomes apparent. This swelling can be localized or can spread through fascial spaces in rare cases. The severity of swelling depends on the immune response, the type of microorganisms involved, and the extent of tissue irritation.

The concept of the postoperative flare up is central to understanding postoperative complications. A flare up is an acute exacerbation of symptoms that develops after treatment and often requires urgent intervention. It is characterized by severe pain, swelling, and sometimes systemic symptoms. Flare ups are more common in teeth with preoperative symptoms, necrotic pulps, or large periapical lesions. Procedural factors such as apical extrusion of debris, incomplete disinfection, or over instrumentation can also contribute to flare ups. Although flare ups are relatively rare, their impact on patient satisfaction and clinician confidence makes them a significant concern.

The epidemiology of postoperative pain provides valuable insight into its clinical significance. Studies show that postoperative discomfort occurs in a significant percentage of patients within the first week after treatment. Most cases involve mild pain, but a smaller percentage experience moderate to severe symptoms. The frequency and intensity of postoperative symptoms vary depending on the type of tooth treated, the presence of preoperative symptoms, and procedural techniques. Understanding these trends helps clinicians anticipate patient responses and prepare appropriate management plans.

In addition to biological mechanisms, procedural technique influences postoperative outcomes. Accurate working length determination, careful use of instruments, proper irrigation protocols, and controlled obturation pressures all reduce the risk of postoperative irritation. Conversely, procedural errors such as overfilling, underfilling, perforations, or missed canals can lead to persistent symptoms. Clinicians must approach each step with attention to detail, recognizing that even small deviations can have significant consequences for postoperative comfort.

Communication with the patient plays an important role in understanding and managing postoperative pain. When patients are informed about the possibility of mild discomfort and understand normal healing patterns, they are better prepared and less anxious when symptoms occur. Clear communication also strengthens trust between the clinician and the patient. When symptoms exceed expected levels, patients feel more comfortable reporting them promptly, allowing clinicians to intervene early.

Understanding postoperative symptoms also supports appropriate use of pharmacologic interventions. Analgesics, anti-inflammatory medications, and antibiotics must be selected based on evidence and clinical need. Overprescribing antibiotics, for example, contributes to resistance and does not address most cases of postoperative discomfort. This chapter prepares the foundation for later discussions on pharmacologic management by emphasizing the importance of accurate diagnosis before prescribing medications.

Another critical aspect of understanding postoperative pain is the recognition of anatomical variations. Teeth with complex root structures, severe curvatures, or accessory canals are more prone to complications. Clinicians must use imaging and careful exploration to identify these variations before treatment. Failure to recognize anatomical challenges increases the risk of incomplete cleaning or unexpected procedural errors.

Finally, understanding postoperative pain and swelling is not only a matter of managing complications but also a reflection of comprehensive care. When clinicians appreciate the biological and procedural factors that influence healing, they approach treatment with greater precision and awareness. This understanding creates better outcomes for patients and supports a more predictable and controlled healing process.

Post obturation pain and swelling are not signs of failure but indications of the biological processes that occur after intervention. By studying these processes, clinicians can refine their techniques, enhance patient outcomes, and contribute to the advancement of non-surgical endodontic practice.

Clinical Case Study 1: Persistent Post Obturation Pain in a Mandibular Molar with Complex Anatomy

A 46 year old teacher presented with dull, constant pain in the lower right first molar that had persisted for more than two months. She reported that the tooth had been restored several times over the years and recently developed sensitivity that progressed into spontaneous pain and difficulty chewing. Clinical examination revealed deep occlusal caries, lingering thermal response, and mild tenderness to percussion. Radiographic assessment suggested irreversible pulpitis with early periapical changes.

The clinician proceeded with non-surgical root canal therapy. After isolation, access was gained and three canals were identified. Cleaning and shaping were completed using a rotary system with copious irrigation. The clinician noted that the mesial canals were particularly narrow and curved, which increased the risk of debris packing. Sodium hypochlorite and EDTA were used throughout the procedure, followed by obturation with gutta percha and sealer. The operator felt the procedure had gone smoothly, and no complications were observed during treatment.

Within twenty four hours, the patient reported significant pain that radiated along the mandible, especially during chewing. She described the discomfort as a deep, pressurized ache. The clinician prescribed analgesics and reassured her that temporary irritation sometimes occurs after treatment. However, by the third day, the patient reported worsening symptoms, including pain during light biting pressure and occasional throbbing at night.

A follow up radiograph was taken, revealing a dense obturation but slight overextension in one of the mesial canals. The clinician suspected that apical trauma or extrusion of debris had triggered an inflammatory response. The patient's history of aggressive inflammation was considered, as she mentioned similar intense reactions after past dental treatments.

Over the next week, analgesics provided partial relief, but the discomfort persisted. The clinician conducted a more detailed evaluation and suspected the presence of an untreated anatomical variant, such as a mid mesial canal. The original access preparation did not show any obvious missed anatomy, but CBCT imaging was recommended to clarify internal morphology. The scan revealed a small but distinct mid mesial canal that contained necrotic remnants and had not been instrumented. This canal served as a reservoir for microbial byproducts that continued to stimulate the periapical tissues, causing persistent pain.

Retreatment was initiated. The existing gutta percha was carefully removed, and the hidden canal was located under magnification. Once accessed, it released necrotic debris with a strong odor, confirming the suspected microbial source. The canals were thoroughly irrigated, activated with ultrasonic agitation, and medicated with calcium hydroxide for one week. At the follow up appointment, the patient reported dramatic improvement. Obturation was completed, and within two days the tooth became comfortable during chewing.

This case demonstrates how anatomical complexity can contribute to persistent postoperative pain even when the visible canals appear well treated. It also highlights the importance of advanced imaging, careful exploration, and a willingness to reassess treatment when symptoms do not resolve as expected. The interaction between microbial persistence and procedural challenges underscores why postoperative pain must always be interpreted with both biological and technical awareness.

Clinical Case Study 2: Acute Post Obturation Swelling Following Debris Extrusion in a Necrotic Tooth

A 39 year old banker presented with a history of swelling and sensitivity in the upper right canine region. The patient reported that the swelling had recurred twice over the past six months and resolved temporarily with antibiotics prescribed elsewhere. Clinical examination revealed that the tooth did not respond to thermal testing, and palpation of the apical area produced mild discomfort. Radiographs showed a well-defined periapical radiolucency extending along the root surface, consistent with chronic periapical periodontitis.

The clinician recommended non-surgical root canal therapy. During treatment, the canal was found to be wide but irregular, with areas of internal resorption. While cleaning and shaping the canal, the clinician encountered heavy necrotic debris. Irrigation was performed with sodium hypochlorite, but due to the large apical diameter and limited control of apical pressure, some irrigant and debris likely passed beyond the apex. The clinician noted slight resistance during irrigation but continued cautiously.

Obturation was performed with warm vertical compaction. The patient was discharged with postoperative instructions and informed that mild discomfort could occur.

By evening, the patient experienced severe throbbing pain and noticed swelling in the upper lip and adjacent vestibule. By the next morning, the swelling had increased significantly, and the patient struggled to chew comfortably. Upon return to the clinic, examination revealed pronounced localized swelling, warmth, and tenderness. There was no fever or systemic involvement at this stage. Radiographs showed a slight extruded mass consistent with debris or excess sealer near the apex.

Based on the timing and symptoms, the clinician diagnosed an acute postoperative flare up triggered by apical extrusion of infected material. The immune system reacted aggressively to the sudden presence of microbial toxins in the periapical tissues, producing a strong inflammatory response characterized by swelling and intense pain.

Management focused on reducing inflammation and controlling pain. The clinician prescribed analgesics and an anti-inflammatory medication. A short course of antibiotics was added because of the advancing swelling and to reduce the risk of space infection. Warm saline rinses were recommended along with instructions to monitor for systemic symptoms.

Over the next forty eight hours, the swelling gradually reduced. By the fourth day, the patient reported significant improvement, and the tissue began returning to normal appearance. At the one week review, the swelling had resolved completely, and the tooth was no longer painful. A follow up radiograph taken three months later showed early signs of bone healing around the periapex.

This case illustrates how even well executed treatment can lead to postoperative complications when biological and mechanical factors interact unfavorably. Apical extrusion of debris, particularly in necrotic teeth, triggers strong tissue reactions because of the high microbial load. The case underscores the importance of gentle irrigation, controlled instrumentation, and awareness of canal anatomy that predisposes to extrusion. It also highlights the need for clinicians to respond promptly and confidently when postoperative swelling occurs.

CHAPTER 2

Etiology of Post Obturation Pain Biological and Mechanical Factors

P ost obturation pain does not arise from a single cause but from a complex interaction of biological, mechanical, microbial, chemical, and patient specific factors. Understanding these sources of irritation is essential for predicting which cases may experience discomfort, for selecting appropriate prevention strategies, and for responding effectively when symptoms occur. Etiology encompasses every event that influences periapical tissues during and after treatment, beginning with the initial diagnosis and continuing through instrumentation, irrigation, obturation, and the immediate healing period. Clinicians who appreciate these contributing factors are better able to reduce complications and improve patient outcomes.

One of the most significant causes of postoperative pain is the presence of persistent microorganisms within the root canal system. Microbes that survive instrumentation and irrigation can produce metabolic byproducts that irritate periapical tissues. The root canal system contains anatomical variations such as lateral canals, accessory canals, apical deltas, fins, and isthmuses that may harbor bacteria even after careful cleaning. These spaces create environments where microorganisms can attach to dentin, form biofilms, and resist chemical penetration. When obturation is completed, these organisms may not be fully eliminated. Their toxins slowly diffuse into the periapical tissues, triggering inflammatory responses characterized by increased vascular permeability, activation of inflammatory mediators, and recruitment of immune cells. These tissue level reactions manifest clinically as postoperative pain, swelling, or both. The challenge is compounded by the fact that biofilm bacteria exhibit increased resistance to irrigants and medicaments. Even small microbial remnants can significantly influence postoperative symptoms.

Another major etiologic factor is apical extrusion of debris, irrigants, or filling materials. During instrumentation, dentinal shavings, necrotic tissue, residual bacteria, and irrigant solution can be pushed beyond the apex if proper control is not maintained. These materials function as foreign irritants and provoke an inflammatory reaction. Extruded debris is particularly problematic in teeth with necrotic pulps, where bacterial loads are high. Once microbial debris enters the periapical space, the immune response becomes amplified because the tissues are directly exposed to pathogens and their toxins. This reaction may lead to acute postoperative pain, and in some cases, swelling or a flare up that requires urgent intervention. Even without microbial content, sterile extrusion of dentin or sealer can irritate apical tissues and trigger painful pressure sensations as the body attempts to break down or isolate foreign material.

Instrument related trauma also plays a considerable role in postoperative symptoms. Over instrumentation, accidental transportation beyond the apex, or repeated mechanical contact with periapical tissues can cause irritation and inflammation. When instruments penetrate beyond the apical constriction, they damage the periodontal ligament and surrounding tissues. These tissues contain sensory nerve fibers that react strongly to mechanical insult. This trauma stimulates production of inflammatory mediators, including prostaglandins and cytokines, which contribute to postoperative hypersensitivity. Additionally, aggressive shaping techniques that create excessive apical enlargement increase the likelihood of tissue irritation because larger apical openings reduce the natural resistance to extrusion and expose periapical tissues to more mechanical stress.

Chemical irritation is another important etiologic category. The solutions used in endodontic therapy, particularly sodium hypochlorite, can cause tissue damage if they pass beyond the apex or come into direct contact with periapical spaces. Sodium hypochlorite accidents are relatively rare, but even small amounts that escape can induce intense inflammatory responses due to their caustic nature. Chlorhexidine, EDTA, and other irrigants can also irritate tissues when introduced inappropriately or used with excessive apical pressure. The type of sealer used during obturation can contribute to postoperative discomfort as well. Certain materials release heat or chemical byproducts during setting, and if extruded or placed directly against apical tissues, they may cause irritation. Bioceramic sealers are generally well tolerated, but other formulations may contain components that provoke inflammation.

Obturation technique contributes significantly to etiology. Techniques that rely on warm vertical compaction introduce heat into the canal, which can affect surrounding tissues if applied excessively. Warm obturation also increases the risk of sealer or gutta percha extrusion due to softened materials flowing beyond the apex. Even cold lateral compaction can cause extrusion if excessive pressure is applied. Obturation also influences postoperative pain through its relationship with apical sealing. Underfilled canals leave microbial remnants unaddressed, allowing persistent irritation. Overfilled canals introduce foreign objects into spaces where tissues are highly sensitive. Both extremes can cause postoperative pain.

Preoperative status of the tooth is one of the strongest predictors of postoperative symptoms. Teeth with necrotic pulps or preexisting periapical lesions have higher rates of postoperative pain because their periapical tissues are already inflamed. When treatment begins in an environment with elevated inflammatory mediators, tissues respond more intensely to mechanical or chemical stimuli. Teeth with symptomatic apical periodontitis have sensitized nerve endings that remain active even after bacterial sources are removed. The reduction of inflammation takes time, and during this transition period, patients may perceive increased pain or pressure.

Occlusal trauma following treatment also contributes to postoperative discomfort. When a tooth that recently underwent instrumentation is subjected to excessive occlusal load, the already sensitized periodontal ligament becomes inflamed. Even minor changes in occlusal contacts can lead to significant discomfort because the tissues surrounding the tooth are not yet stable. High occlusion is a common but often overlooked contributor to postoperative pain, especially when the tooth receives a permanent or temporary restoration that unintentionally alters bite dynamics.

Host factors also influence postoperative responses. The patient's immune system, pain threshold, and systemic health conditions shape how symptoms develop. Individuals with strong inflammatory responses may experience more pronounced pain or swelling even when treatment is technically sound. Conditions such as diabetes, immune compromise, and anxiety can alter perception of pain and tissue healing speed. Medications the patient is taking, including antihypertensives, anticoagulants, or immunosuppressants, may also influence tissue responses. These factors explain why two patients with identical treatment experiences may report very different postoperative outcomes.

Coronal leakage contributes to postoperative pain when bacterial contamination occurs soon after treatment. If the temporary or permanent restoration is inadequate, oral fluids containing bacteria may infiltrate the canal system and reach the periapical tissues. This leads to renewed microbial irritation and can mimic the pain associated with untreated canals or persistent infection. Proper restoration and adequate sealing are critical in preventing reinfection and the associated postoperative symptoms.

The biological mechanisms that underlie postoperative pain are rooted in the inflammatory response. When tissues experience irritation, damaged cells release mediators such as bradykinin, prostaglandins, and histamine. These substances increase blood flow, promote fluid movement into tissues, and sensitize nerve fibers. Sensitized nerves transmit pain signals more readily, leading to heightened perception of discomfort. Swelling occurs as fluid accumulates due to increased vascular permeability. In severe cases, pressure from fluid buildup triggers additional pain and may limit function. Understanding these reactions underscores that postoperative pain is not simply a reflection of procedural error but often the natural result of tissue inflammation and healing.

A deeper look at microbial etiology reveals that different species of bacteria contribute differently to postoperative symptoms. Gram negative anaerobes, which commonly inhabit necrotic pulp systems, release endotoxins that are highly inflammatory. These toxins can penetrate dentinal tubules and existing accessory canals even after thorough cleaning. Facultative anaerobes may also persist in difficult to reach areas and stimulate inflammation. The severity of postoperative symptoms often depends on the concentration and type of bacteria present before treatment. Teeth with chronic infections may contain bacteria that have adapted to the canal environment and possess strong biofilm structures. These biofilms can resist instrumentation, irrigation, and medicaments, increasing the likelihood of postoperative irritation.

Mechanical etiology also includes procedural factors such as incomplete removal of pulp tissue. If remnants of inflamed or necrotic tissue remain within the canal system, the body continues to respond to this material as an irritant. This response may lead to a prolonged postoperative course. In addition, failure to address anatomical complexity increases the chances of untreated areas becoming sources of persistent irritation. The clinician's ability to recognize and navigate anatomical variations plays a significant role in minimizing postoperative symptoms.

Another contributor to postoperative pain is air entrapment within the canal or periapical tissues. When instruments or irrigants introduce air bubbles that become trapped, they can exert pressure on sensitive tissues. Although rare, this phenomenon can cause pain when the patient bites or applies pressure to the tooth. Proper irrigation techniques that avoid injecting air prevent this problem.

In some cases, postoperative pain may be the result of healing processes rather than pathological irritation. As periapical inflammation resolves, tissues undergo a period of remodeling. During this process, patients may experience intermittent sensitivity or mild discomfort. Recognizing this healing pattern helps clinicians provide appropriate reassurance and avoid unnecessary intervention.

Altogether, the etiology of post obturation pain is a multifaceted topic influenced by microbial, mechanical, chemical, anatomical, and patient related variables. Understanding these factors equips clinicians to anticipate complications, modify techniques, and respond effectively when symptoms arise. By appreciating the biological context in which endodontic treatment occurs, practitioners can foster a more predictable and comfortable healing environment for their patients.

2.1 Influence of Irrigation Dynamics and Fluid Mechanics on Post Obturation Pain

Irrigation is a cornerstone of successful endodontic therapy, but the manner in which irrigants move within the canal system has profound implications for postoperative comfort. Irrigation dynamics determine how effectively debris is removed, how deeply solutions penetrate into anatomical irregularities, and how much pressure is exerted toward the apical region. All of these factors contribute to the likelihood of irritation after obturation.

The behavior of irrigating solutions within the canal is governed by principles of fluid mechanics. When irrigants are delivered with excessive force or inserted too deeply into the canal, they generate apical pressure that can displace debris or solution beyond the apex. Even a minor extrusion of sodium hypochlorite or chlorhexidine can provoke significant periapical inflammation because these solutions are not biocompatible when they leave the confines of the canal. Irritant effects include tissue necrosis, vascular leakage, and activation of inflammatory pathways that intensify postoperative pain.

Another important factor is the presence of vapor lock in the apical third. Vapor lock is a phenomenon where air becomes trapped in the apical portion of the canal, preventing irrigants from reaching the deepest areas. When the canal contains air pockets, irrigants are unable to contact and dissolve necrotic tissue or reach microbial biofilms. Persistent debris and microorganisms left behind after instrumentation become sources of postoperative irritation.

Activation systems, including ultrasonic and sonic devices, influence irrigation dynamics by disrupting air entrapment and enhancing irrigant flow. While these systems improve disinfection, they can also increase the risk of extrusion when not used with caution. Continuous irrigation movement generates acoustic streaming and cavitation, which can push debris toward the apex if the canal is not properly shaped. Understanding these physical interactions helps clinicians adjust irrigation techniques to minimize postoperative complications while optimizing cleaning efficiency.

The heat generated by activated irrigation also has a role in postoperative sensitivity. Increased temperature enhances the effectiveness of sodium hypochlorite in dissolving tissue, but when temperature rises near the apical region, the surrounding tissues may react with increased sensitivity. Although such cases are uncommon, they illustrate how the physics of irrigation interacts with biological structures in ways that influence postoperative outcomes.

By appreciating the relationship between irrigation dynamics and postoperative pain, clinicians can refine their techniques through cautious needle placement, gentle pressure, improved activation methods, and thorough canal shaping. This careful approach reduces the likelihood of periapical irritation and improves overall treatment predictability.

2.2 Material Biocompatibility and Tissue Response as Etiologic Factors in Post Obturation Pain

The materials used during obturation play a crucial role in determining the biological response that follows treatment. Although many modern endodontic materials are designed with biocompatibility in mind, variations in chemical composition, setting reactions, and interaction with tissues all influence the degree of postoperative discomfort that patients may experience. Understanding how these materials behave biologically provides deeper insight into why some patients develop symptoms even when treatment appears technically successful.

Gutta percha is generally well tolerated by periapical tissues, but sealer formulations vary significantly in their biocompatibility. Traditional resin based sealers may release monomers or setting byproducts that can irritate tissues when extruded beyond the apex. Zinc oxide eugenol sealers release eugenol, a compound known to cause inflammatory reactions in sensitive tissues. Calcium hydroxide based sealers promote healing but may create initial irritation due to their alkalinity. Bioceramic sealers tend to be well accepted, but their flowability can lead to extrusion in cases with large apical diameters, resulting in foreign body reactions.

The process of obturation itself involves mechanical pressure that can push sealer or gutta percha beyond the apical confines. Even biocompatible materials may trigger inflammation simply because they occupy spaces meant for vascular and connective tissues. The body responds to extruded material by attempting to encapsulate or resorb it. During this period, immune cells release mediators that cause pain, swelling, or tenderness.

Thermal obturation techniques further influence tissue response. Warm vertical compaction uses elevated temperatures to soften gutta percha, allowing it to flow into canal irregularities. However, when heat is applied near the apex, it can influence the surrounding tissues by raising their temperature slightly. Although this temperature rise rarely causes direct damage, it may contribute to temporary postoperative sensitivity. The interaction of heat with sealer setting reactions can also influence how materials behave once they reach periapical areas.

Material induced inflammation may also occur when sealer interacts with moisture in the canal, especially if the canal was not adequately dried. Moisture affects setting properties and may lead to incomplete polymerization of certain sealers. In such cases, unset particles or unstable chemical components may leak into surrounding tissues, causing irritation.

In addition, the long term presence of extruded sealer can contribute to delayed healing. Studies reveal that some extruded materials persist for years and appear radiographically unchanged. Even when they are not actively harmful, their presence can maintain a mild inflammatory response that manifests intermittently as tenderness or pressure sensitivity.

This response often resolves naturally, but in other cases, persistent irritation requires surgical intervention.

Material biocompatibility is therefore a significant etiologic factor in postoperative discomfort. The choice of sealer, the obturation technique, the apical size, and the management of canal moisture all combine to influence how tissues react after treatment. Clinicians who understand these interactions are better able to predict patient outcomes and minimize irritation by selecting appropriate materials and handling them carefully.

CHAPTER 3

Pathophysiology of Post Obturation Complications

U nderstanding the pathophysiology behind post obturation pain and swelling requires a close examination of the biological events that unfold within the periapical tissues following root canal treatment. These events are influenced by microbial remnants, mechanical stimuli, chemical irritants, immune response patterns, and neurophysiologic mechanisms that determine how the body interprets and reacts to irritation. While postoperative symptoms may appear sudden or unpredictable, they result from a sequence of tissue level reactions that reflect the body's attempt to defend, repair, or regulate damaged areas. A thorough understanding of these processes allows clinicians to anticipate complications, explain symptoms accurately to patients, and select evidence based interventions.

At the core of postoperative discomfort is inflammation, which is the body's natural response to injury or irritation. Inflammation begins immediately when tissues are disturbed by instrumentation or exposed to microbial byproducts. Damaged cells release mediators such as histamine, prostaglandins, serotonin, and bradykinin. These substances initiate vasodilation, increase blood flow, and make vascular walls more permeable. As fluid exits the vessels and accumulates within the surrounding tissues, swelling develops. Meanwhile, immune cells migrate to the site of irritation, where they attempt to neutralize harmful substances. The resulting cascade of events produces pressure, temperature changes, and chemical signals that stimulate sensory nerve endings, leading to pain.

The presence of microbial components intensifies this process significantly. Even after thorough cleaning, traces of bacterial biofilm, endotoxins, or cell wall fragments may remain within canal spaces or dentinal tubules. These remnants activate toll like receptors on immune cells, which recognize microbial molecules and initiate a strong inflammatory response. The periapical environment becomes rich in cytokines such as interleukin one, interleukin six, and tumor necrosis factor alpha. These mediators amplify inflammation by increasing vascular dilation, enhancing leukocyte activity, and maintaining the sensitization of nociceptors. Because these reactions evolve in a confined space within the periapical region, even minor increases in cellular activity can produce significant pain.

Neurogenic inflammation also contributes to postoperative symptoms. Nerve fibers within the periodontal ligament and apical tissues release neuropeptides such as substance P and calcitonin gene related peptide when stimulated by mechanical or chemical irritants. These neuropeptides further enhance vascular permeability and vasodilation, creating a feedback loop that intensifies inflammation. Neurogenic inflammation is particularly important in explaining why some patients experience severe postoperative pain even when radiographs appear normal. The nervous system's reaction to tissue injury can be disproportionately intense, especially in individuals with heightened pain sensitivity.

Another component of pathophysiology is the role of pressure dynamics within the periapical region. During obturation, materials may introduce slight pressure against apical tissues. In cases where debris or fluid extrudes beyond the apex, the confined periapical space becomes a site of dramatic pressure changes. Increased interstitial pressure compresses nerve fibers and contributes to throbbing sensations that worsen with bending, chewing, or lying down. If the inflammatory process is severe, fluid accumulation may exceed the tissue's ability to regulate pressure, resulting in visible swelling. This accumulation begins with transudate but may progress to exudate if cellular activity and vascular permeability increase further.

Chemical irritation from irrigants or sealers contributes another dimension to pathophysiology. Sodium hypochlorite, a commonly used irrigant, is highly effective inside the canal but harmful to living tissues if it escapes. Even minimal exposure causes tissue necrosis, induces rapid edema, and activates acute inflammatory pathways. The surrounding tissues respond with intense pain due to direct chemical injury combined with secondary inflammation. Sealer materials can also cause irritation before they fully set. Resin based sealers may release monomers, while certain zinc oxide formulations release eugenol, which can irritate nerve endings and connective tissue. Calcium hydroxide sealers produce an alkaline environment that can initially stimulate inflammation before promoting healing.

Another important mechanism is the activation of the complement system. Microbial antigens or tissue damage triggers complement proteins that promote chemotaxis, enhance phagocyte activity, and increase vascular permeability. These reactions are part of the innate immune response and can significantly heighten inflammation in the immediate postoperative period. The complement cascade is especially active in teeth with preexisting periapical lesions because chronic infection primes the immune system, making it more reactive to postoperative stimuli.

Pathophysiology also involves the interaction of inflammatory mediators with nociceptors. Prostaglandins sensitize nerve fibers by lowering their activation threshold, which makes them more responsive to stimuli. Bradykinin stimulates pain directly by binding to receptors on nociceptors. These mechanisms explain why postoperative pain may appear exaggerated compared to the actual level of tissue damage. In sensitized tissues, even mild pressure or temperature changes can produce intense pain signals. This phenomenon is known as hyperalgesia. In some cases, allodynia may occur, where non painful stimuli such as tapping or chewing produce significant discomfort.

The periapical tissues undergo complex cellular activity during the early stages of healing. Neutrophils arrive first and attempt to eliminate irritants. Their presence is essential but can contribute to tissue breakdown because they release enzymes that degrade damaged material. Macrophages follow and play a larger role in orchestrating healing. They remove debris, regulate inflammation, and stimulate fibroblasts that rebuild tissue. However, when microbial remnants persist, macrophages continue to release pro inflammatory cytokines, prolonging pain and delaying healing. Chronic inflammation may develop if the irritant is not eliminated, resulting in intermittent postoperative symptoms.

Another critical aspect of pathophysiology involves the lymphatic system. The periapical region has limited lymphatic drainage, which means fluid and inflammatory mediators may accumulate more easily. Poor drainage prolongs swelling and increases the duration of pain. This limited clearance capacity explains why postoperative swelling may take several days to resolve even when treatment has successfully eliminated the source of irritation.

In cases of acute flare ups, pathophysiology becomes more dramatic. A flare up represents a significant imbalance between microbial load, immune response, and tissue stability. Rapid bacterial proliferation or sudden release of toxins overwhelms local tissues, creating intense inflammation. The immune system responds aggressively, but because the canal is sealed, pressure may build rapidly. This pressure further irritates nerve fibers and may lead to spreading swelling. Understanding flare ups through the lens of pathophysiology helps clinicians manage them calmly. They represent a biological crisis rather than a procedural error, although procedural factors may contribute.

Thermal changes within the canal also influence postoperative symptoms. Heat from warm obturation may affect dentinal fluid movement and thermal sensitivity. Although these effects are usually transient, they contribute to early postoperative discomfort. As the sealer sets and the thermal stress subsides, symptoms typically diminish.

The relationship between systemic health and pathophysiologic responses must also be considered. Patients with diabetes, autoimmune disorders, cardiovascular disease, or chronic inflammatory conditions may exhibit exaggerated or prolonged responses. Their immune regulation differs from that of healthy individuals, altering healing speed and pain perception. Medications such as anticoagulants, corticosteroids, and antihypertensives may influence tissue reactions and vascular responses.

Finally, the pathophysiology of postoperative complications teaches an important clinical lesson. Endodontic treatment is not simply a mechanical procedure but a biological one. Every action taken within the canal interacts with living tissues that react in ways that are predictable when understood but difficult to manage when ignored. By recognizing the underlying biological processes, clinicians can better anticipate complications, tailor pain management strategies, and communicate clearly with patients about what to expect during healing.

3.1 The Role of Periapical Vascular Changes in Post Obturation Pain

Periapical tissues depend heavily on a stable microvascular network to regulate healing after endodontic treatment. When irritation occurs, the first physiological response involves changes in local blood flow. Blood vessels in the periodontal ligament and periapical region undergo vasodilation triggered by inflammatory mediators such as histamine, prostaglandins, and nitric oxide. Vasodilation increases blood supply to the affected area, allowing immune cells and plasma proteins to reach the site of irritation. While this process is essential for defense and repair, it also introduces conditions that contribute to pain.

Increased vascular permeability is one of the earliest and most significant changes. As endothelial cells within vessel walls widen their junctions under the influence of chemical mediators, fluid and proteins escape into the surrounding tissues. This movement of fluid creates interstitial swelling, which increases pressure within the confined space surrounding the root apex. Periapical tissues, particularly in multi rooted teeth, have limited capacity to expand because they are bordered by bone. As pressure builds, nerve fibers within the periodontal ligament become compressed and sensitized, giving rise to throbbing or pulsating pain.

When microbial byproducts or extruded debris stimulate strong inflammatory responses, blood vessels may become engorged and congested. Congestion limits venous return and further increases hydrostatic pressure in the area. This vascular stagnation prolongs inflammation and contributes to a cycle of persistent discomfort. The degree of pain a patient experiences often reflects the intensity of vascular changes rather than the size of the periapical lesion. Even small lesions can produce significant pain if vascular congestion is severe.

The lymphatic system plays a complementary but equally important role. Lymphatic vessels help clear excess fluid and inflammatory mediators from the periapical region. However, the lymphatic network in dental tissues is not robust, and when inflammatory load becomes overwhelming, clearance is inefficient. The result is sustained swelling and prolonged sensitivity. These vascular and lymphatic dynamics illustrate why some patients recover quickly while others require several days for symptoms to resolve.

Understanding these microvascular changes helps clinicians anticipate postoperative discomfort and tailor their management strategies. For example, anti-inflammatory medications work by reducing vascular dilation and permeability, thereby alleviating pressure and pain. Recognizing the vascular basis of pain underscores the importance of controlling procedural irritation and microbial load during treatment.

3.2 Neurophysiological Processing of Pain in Post Obturation Complications

Pain perception is not solely a result of local tissue injury. It is shaped by complex neurophysiological mechanisms that begin in the periapical tissues and extend to the central nervous system. Each nociceptor, or pain receptor, located in the periodontal ligament and apical tissues transmits signals through the trigeminal nerve to higher processing centers in the brain. The intensity and quality of postoperative pain depend on how these signals are generated, transmitted, and interpreted.

During root canal therapy, mechanical and chemical stimuli activate nociceptors directly. When inflammatory mediators such as prostaglandins and bradykinin accumulate, they dramatically lower the activation threshold of these nerve endings. This sensitization explains why normal biting pressure may cause discomfort after treatment. Nociceptors fire more rapidly and with greater intensity in sensitized tissues, producing heightened pain responses known as hyperalgesia.

In some cases, the nervous system becomes so sensitized that non painful stimuli trigger pain, a phenomenon known as allodynia. For example, tapping the tooth lightly or simply touching adjacent tissues may produce discomfort. This response occurs because persistent inflammation alters the way sensory pathways process information. Sensitization may occur at the peripheral level within the tissues or centrally within the spinal nucleus of the trigeminal nerve.

Central sensitization is particularly important in understanding patients who report severe postoperative pain that seems disproportionate to clinical findings. When neurons in the trigeminal nucleus become hyperresponsive due to ongoing inflammatory input, they amplify signals, creating an exaggerated perception of pain. This mechanism may persist even after local tissues begin to heal, leading to prolonged discomfort.

Another component of neurophysiology involves the release of neuropeptides such as substance P and calcitonin gene related peptide. These neuropeptides contribute to both pain and inflammation. Substance P promotes vasodilation, enhances vascular permeability, and facilitates communication between immune cells and nerve fibers. Calcitonin gene related peptide increases blood flow and can prolong inflammatory reactions. Together, these neuropeptides create a cycle in which pain stimulates inflammation and inflammation stimulates pain.

Clinicians benefit from understanding these processes because they explain why postoperative pain varies widely among individuals and why some patients require more support than others. Neurophysiologic mechanisms also justify the use of medications that modulate nerve activity, such as non-steroidal anti-inflammatory drugs and corticosteroids. By targeting the mediators that influence nerve sensitization, these medications reduce both pain and inflammation.

3.3 Cellular Interactions and Immune System Dynamics in Post Obturation Swelling

The immune system plays a decisive role in shaping postoperative outcomes. Once irritation occurs in the periapical region, immune cells migrate to the site and interact in a coordinated effort to neutralize irritants and support healing. These interactions define the degree of swelling, the intensity of pain, and the speed of recovery.

Neutrophils are the first responders during acute inflammation. Their arrival is rapid and mediated by chemical signals released by damaged cells and microbial fragments. Neutrophils release enzymes such as elastase and collagenase to break down debris and microorganisms. However, these enzymes also affect the surrounding tissues, sometimes intensifying inflammation. Their activity contributes to the internal swelling that occurs immediately after obturation in some patients.

Macrophages arrive later and assume a more controlled role. They engulf debris, regulate inflammatory activity, and secrete cytokines that influence the next phase of healing. When bacterial remnants persist, macrophages remain in a heightened state of activation, continuously releasing inflammatory mediators. This prolonged activity contributes to chronic postoperative discomfort. Macrophages also stimulate fibroblasts to begin tissue repair, but if irritants remain, this process becomes inefficient, leading to periods of recurring tenderness.

Lymphocytes may become involved when the immune system identifies persistent antigens. Their presence indicates a more chronic or deep seated inflammatory environment. In such cases, swelling may occur intermittently as the immune system attempts to control microbial remnants. Chronic apical periodontitis is the result of these long term interactions, and postoperative symptoms may continue until the irritant is eliminated through retreatment or surgical intervention.

The complement system represents another important immune mechanism. Complement proteins bind to microbial antigens and activate a chain of biochemical reactions that enhance inflammation. These reactions stimulate phagocytes, promote chemotaxis, and increase vascular permeability. In severe postoperative flare ups, complement activation contributes to dramatic swelling and pain.

Understanding these cellular interactions helps clinicians predict which teeth are more prone to postoperative symptoms. Teeth with necrotic pulps, longstanding infections, or large lesions often harbor microorganisms that challenge the immune system, making postoperative inflammation stronger and more prolonged. Effective management requires reducing microbial load and minimizing further tissue irritation during treatment.

CHAPTER 4

Clinical Assessment and Diagnostic Framework for Post Obturation Symptoms

Accurate clinical assessment is essential for understanding and managing post obturation pain and swelling. Although these symptoms are common, they vary widely in severity, duration, and underlying cause. Some discomfort is a normal part of tissue healing, while other presentations signal complications that require immediate attention. The challenge for clinicians is distinguishing expected postoperative reactions from pathological conditions that demand intervention. This requires a systematic diagnostic approach grounded in knowledge of endodontic biology, procedural influences, and patient specific factors.

The first step in assessment is obtaining a detailed history of the patient's symptoms. Clinicians must ask when the pain began, how it has changed over time, and what activities exacerbate or relieve it. Pain that begins within the first twenty four to forty eight hours after treatment is typically consistent with normal postoperative inflammation. However, pain that intensifies over several days or begins after an initial period of comfort may indicate microbial activity or procedural complications. Questions about chewing, biting, spontaneous pain, night pain, and thermal sensitivity help build a clearer clinical picture. Swelling, fever, or a feeling of pressure also provide important diagnostic clues.

Understanding the preoperative condition of the tooth is critical. Teeth that had symptomatic apical periodontitis, necrotic pulps, or large periapical lesions before treatment are more likely to exhibit postoperative discomfort. These tissues were already inflamed and sensitized before the procedure, and their healing process requires time. Knowing the initial diagnosis helps clinicians avoid misinterpreting expected postoperative sensitivity as treatment failure. In contrast, a tooth that was asymptomatic before treatment but develops intense postoperative pain warrants closer evaluation.

Clinical examination begins with visual inspection of the surrounding soft tissues. Swelling, redness, or fluctuation suggests that inflammation has progressed beyond the tooth itself. Diffuse swelling that extends into vestibular or facial spaces may indicate that the inflammatory response has created pressure that exceeds normal tissue limits. Lack of swelling does not rule out a significant problem, but its presence provides valuable diagnostic insight. Intraoral swelling that is firm and tender usually reflects significant inflammatory edema, while swelling that feels fluctuant may indicate the presence of exudate.

Percussion testing remains a sensitive indicator of periapical inflammation. A tooth that produces discomfort on percussion typically has irritated periodontal ligament fibers. Mild tenderness is common after treatment, but sharp or intense pain on tapping suggests active inflammation or microbial involvement. Palpation over the apical region helps identify swelling, sensitivity, and pressure. A firm tender area often reflects edema, while a soft compressible area may reflect the development of an abscess.

Bite testing provides additional information. Many patients experience discomfort during chewing because of inflammation in the periodontal ligament. However, sharp localized pain during bite testing may indicate a cracked tooth or high occlusion. Occlusal assessment is essential because minor discrepancies can dramatically increase postoperative discomfort. A recently treated tooth may not tolerate excess occlusal load due to heightened sensitivity in the periodontal ligament.

Thermal testing is sometimes helpful but must be interpreted cautiously, as the pulp has been removed. Thermal sensitivity after root canal therapy may indicate irritation of periodontal structures rather than pulpal pathology. Cold sensitivity in a tooth that has undergone therapy can occur if the tooth structure transmits temperature changes to inflamed periodontal tissues.

Radiographic evaluation plays a central role in diagnosing postoperative complications. A standard periapical radiograph allows clinicians to assess the quality of obturation, the presence of voids, the length of the filling material, and the relationship of the obturation to anatomical structures. Overextension of sealer or gutta percha beyond the apex can irritate tissues and contribute to postoperative pain. Underfilled canals may harbor bacteria that continue to stimulate inflammation. Missed canals or anatomical variations can also be identified radiographically, although subtle variations may require more advanced imaging.

Cone beam computed tomography offers superior visualization of anatomical complexity, hidden canals, and subtle periapical changes. It allows clinicians to identify untreated anatomy, fractures, resorption, and small periapical lesions that may not be visible on two dimensional radiographs. In the context of postoperative symptoms, CBCT is invaluable when patients report persistent pain despite technically adequate treatment.

Pain scales and symptom characterization support diagnostic accuracy. Asking patients to rate pain intensity on a numerical scale from zero to ten allows clinicians to track progress objectively. Describing the quality of pain also provides important clues. Throbbing or pulsating pain often reflects pressure or vascular changes, while sharp pain may indicate occlusal trauma or mechanical irritation. Dull aching pain can result from lingering inflammation or microbial persistence.

Differential diagnosis is essential because postoperative symptoms may mimic other dental or nondental conditions. For example, occlusal trauma can present with symptoms similar to periapical inflammation. Fractures, periodontal disease, and referred pain from adjacent structures must also be considered. A cracked tooth may cause characteristic pain during release of biting pressure, while periodontal abscesses may present with localized swelling and tenderness that differ from endodontically related inflammation. Nonodontogenic pain originating from muscles, nerves, or sinus tissues may complicate diagnosis, especially in maxillary teeth.

Assessing the timeline of symptoms helps determine whether the condition is resolving or worsening. Normal postoperative pain gradually decreases over time. Pain that intensifies or becomes more frequent is concerning. Swelling that develops several days after treatment or recurs after a period of remission indicates microbial involvement and requires immediate attention. When symptoms escalate rapidly, a postoperative flare up is likely, and prompt management is necessary.

The presence or absence of systemic symptoms also informs diagnosis. Fever, malaise, or lymph node tenderness may indicate that the inflammatory process has progressed beyond localized tissues. Although systemic involvement is uncommon after endodontic treatment, recognizing these signs ensures timely intervention.

Another diagnostic consideration involves understanding the influence of patient specific variables. Some individuals experience stronger inflammatory responses due to genetic predisposition, immune system characteristics, or medical conditions. A history of exaggerated responses to dental treatment or slow healing patterns suggests that postoperative symptoms may be more pronounced even when treatment is adequate. Medications such as bisphosphonates, corticosteroids, and anticoagulants can influence tissue response and must be considered during diagnosis.

Communication with the patient is a key component of assessment. Listening carefully to how the patient describes the pain and what they believe may be causing it provides insights into symptom interpretation. Patients who feel heard are more likely to provide accurate descriptions and adhere to recommended interventions. Clear explanation of expected healing patterns also prevents unnecessary anxiety and supports more accurate reporting of abnormal symptoms.

Integrating all diagnostic information allows clinicians to classify postoperative symptoms as expected healing, heightened inflammatory response, early complication, or severe complication requiring urgent management. For instance, mild tenderness without swelling signals expected inflammation.

Persistent pain with no improvement may indicate microbial survival. Severe pain with swelling often represents a flare up. Each classification guides treatment decisions and determines whether observation, pharmacologic support, occlusal adjustment, retreatment, drainage, or referral is appropriate.

Diagnostic accuracy is strengthened when clinicians approach each case with a structured framework rather than relying on assumptions. Postoperative symptoms are shaped by microbial, mechanical, and biological factors that are not always visible. Careful assessment ensures that clinicians identify the true cause of discomfort and intervene appropriately. This protects patients, preserves tooth structure, and improves long term outcomes.

The goal of clinical assessment is not only to identify complications but also to support patient confidence and provide reassurance. Clear diagnosis and timely action reduce anxiety and prevent the escalation of symptoms. By maintaining a disciplined diagnostic approach grounded in evidence and clinical experience, clinicians can manage postoperative symptoms with accuracy and compassion.

Case Study 1: Differentiating Normal Postoperative Sensitivity from an Early Complication in a Mandibular First Molar

A 35 year old accountant presented for follow up forty eight hours after root canal therapy on the lower right first molar. Before treatment, the tooth had been diagnosed with symptomatic irreversible pulpitis and normal periapical tissues.

The clinician performed a single visit procedure, completing cleaning, shaping, and obturation without any intraoperative complications. The patient left the clinic comfortable and was informed that some tenderness could occur during the early healing period.

Two days later, the patient returned with concerns about persistent discomfort. He described the pain as a mild but noticeable pressure sensation during chewing. He denied any spontaneous pain or nighttime episodes. He also had no swelling, fever, bad taste, or sensitivity to temperature. His primary concern was that the pain seemed unchanged since the day after treatment.

The clinician began assessment by taking a detailed history. The patient reported that the discomfort only occurred when chewing on harder foods, such as meat or nuts. He did not experience pain when at rest. This pattern suggested a localized response at the level of the periodontal ligament rather than active infection. The clinician also asked about changes in the quality of pain. The patient noted no progression of symptoms and no new sensations such as throbbing or pulsation.

Clinical examination began with visual inspection. Soft tissues around the treated tooth appeared normal, with no redness or swelling. There was no elevation of the floor of the mouth or facial asymmetry. Palpation over the apical region produced mild tenderness, which aligned with expected inflammatory response following instrumentation.

Percussion testing revealed slight discomfort compared to adjacent teeth, but the response was not sharp or intense. This suggested inflammation of the periodontal ligament rather than severe irritation or microbial activity. Bite testing using a bite stick revealed more distinct tenderness when applying force to the mesiobuccal cusp, indicating that occlusal loading may have been a contributing factor. Thermal tests were not helpful because the tooth had already been extirpated.

Radiographic examination showed a well condensed obturation with no signs of overfilling, voids, or missed canals. The periodontal ligament space appeared slightly widened, consistent with postoperative inflammation. There were no signs of periapical radiolucency or progressive pathology.

Based on the combination of stable symptoms, normal radiographic findings, and the absence of swelling or systemic features, the clinician diagnosed normal postoperative sensitivity compounded by mild occlusal trauma. An occlusal adjustment was performed to relieve excessive force on the treated tooth. The patient was advised to continue using anti-inflammatory medication for another twenty four to forty eight hours and to avoid chewing hard foods on that side temporarily.

To clarify canal morphology, the clinician ordered a cone beam computed tomography scan. The CBCT confirmed the presence of an untreated MB2 canal with a separate orifice and apical exit. The untreated canal contained radiopaque debris and likely harbored persistent microorganisms. This anatomical complexity had not been identified during the initial treatment due to limited visibility in the access cavity.

The clinician diagnosed a postoperative flare up triggered by microbial activity within the untreated canal. The presence of swelling and severe pain indicated an active inflammatory response that required immediate management. The clinician relieved occlusion to reduce periodontal ligament stress, prescribed analgesics, and initiated antibiotic therapy due to the presence of spreading inflammation.

Retreatment was scheduled for the next day. Under magnification, the clinician located the MB2 canal, instrumented it thoroughly, and irrigated it with activated sodium hypochlorite. Calcium hydroxide was placed to reduce microbial load and stabilize the periapical tissues. The patient experienced rapid improvement within forty eight hours. Swelling decreased significantly, and pain became manageable with mild analgesics. Final obturation was completed one week later.

This case demonstrates how missed anatomy can lead to significant postoperative complications and highlights the importance of systematic assessment. Without careful evaluation, the clinician might have mistaken the symptoms for normal postoperative pain or solely attributed them to a flare up without identifying the true cause. CBCT imaging and structured clinical reasoning were essential for accurate diagnosis and successful resolution.

CHAPTER 5

Evidence Based Prevention Strategies for Post Obturation Pain and Swelling

Prevention of post obturation complications begins long before the canal is filled. It requires understanding the biological triggers of postoperative reactions and applying clinical strategies that reduce irritation, minimize microbial load, and protect periapical tissues from unnecessary stress. Successful prevention is built on deliberate diagnostic reasoning, precise technique, and continuous evaluation throughout treatment. Although postoperative discomfort can never be eliminated completely, evidence based protocols substantially reduce both its frequency and severity.

The foundation of prevention lies in accurate diagnosis and case selection. Before beginning treatment, clinicians must determine whether the case involves irreversible pulpitis, necrotic pulp, acute apical abscess, chronic periapical pathology, or a combination of these conditions. Necrotic teeth and teeth with symptomatic apical periodontitis are more prone to postoperative complications because they harbor higher microbial loads and exhibit active inflammation in periapical tissues. When clinicians identify high risk cases early, they can modify their protocols by incorporating staged treatment, intracanal medicaments, or enhanced irrigation techniques.

Establishing proper working length is one of the most effective ways to prevent postoperative pain. Working beyond the apical constriction increases the risk of instrumenting periapical tissues, extruding debris, or irritating sensitive structures. Conversely, under instrumentation leaves microbial reservoirs intact. The use of electronic apex locators combined with radiographic verification offers the most accurate determination of canal length. This dual approach reduces the likelihood of apical transportation and minimizes trauma that contributes to postoperative inflammation.

Instrumentation technique plays a central role in prevention. Evidence shows that crown down and hybrid shaping techniques reduce apical debris extrusion compared to traditional step back methods. Rotary and reciprocating systems are designed to limit debris compaction in the apical region, but this advantage is only realized when clinicians maintain light apical pressure and ensure patency without forcing instruments beyond the apex. Glide path preparation reduces stress on the canal walls and prevents ledging, transportation, and instrument separation, all of which can cause tissue irritation that contributes to postoperative pain.

Irrigation protocols have a profound influence on prevention. Irrigants must be delivered in a manner that maximizes antimicrobial effectiveness while minimizing apical pressure. Sodium hypochlorite remains the most important irrigant due to its ability to dissolve organic tissue, disrupt biofilms, and neutralize bacterial toxins. However, the concentration, temperature, and method of activation determine how effectively it reaches complex anatomical areas. Using side venting needles, maintaining a safe distance from the apex, and applying gentle agitation reduce the risk of extrusion. Supplementary irrigants such as EDTA remove the inorganic smear layer, improving penetration of disinfecting agents into dentinal tubules. Final irrigation protocols that incorporate activation with ultrasonic or passive sonic systems enhance cleaning while lowering the risk of persistent microbial irritation.

Another essential preventive strategy is controlling the apical size. Excessive enlargement of the apical canal increases the likelihood of extrusion during both instrumentation and obturation. Although adequate shaping is needed to facilitate irrigation and obturation, the apical constriction must be preserved whenever possible. Balanced apical enlargement allows irrigants to penetrate more effectively while maintaining a natural barrier that protects periapical tissues.

Effective prevention also includes managing intracanal microbial load. In cases of necrotic pulp or symptomatic apical periodontitis, placing an intracanal medicament such as calcium hydroxide significantly reduces postoperative symptoms. Calcium hydroxide has antimicrobial, anti inflammatory, and tissue stabilizing properties that complement mechanical cleaning. When used for one to two weeks, it reduces bacterial populations and neutralizes endotoxins that would otherwise stimulate postoperative inflammation.

Obturation technique also influences preventive success. Warm vertical compaction must be used with careful control to avoid excessive pressure that can extrude gutta percha or sealer. Cold lateral compaction requires gentle strokes to prevent lateral forces from driving material through accessory canals or the apical foramen. Selecting a biocompatible sealer that forms a strong seal without irritating tissues contributes to long term comfort. Clinicians must ensure that canals are dried appropriately because moisture can alter sealer behavior and lead to incomplete polymerization, which increases the risk of irritation.

Occlusal reduction is another important evidence based strategy for preventing postoperative pain. Teeth undergoing endodontic treatment often have inflamed periodontal ligaments and may not tolerate normal occlusal loading immediately after treatment. Reducing occlusion, especially in teeth that were painful upon biting before treatment, decreases postoperative discomfort significantly. This step is particularly beneficial in molars and premolars where occlusal forces are greatest.

Prevention also involves managing the patient's systemic and local conditions. Patients with compromised immune systems, diabetes, chronic inflammatory disorders, or heightened anxiety may experience stronger postoperative responses. For these individuals, staged treatment, careful monitoring, and enhanced pain management strategies can reduce complications. Communicating clearly with patients about what to expect during healing reduces anxiety and prevents misinterpretation of normal symptoms as complications.

Coronal sealing remains a vital preventive measure. Once the canal is obturated, bacteria from the oral cavity must be prevented from reentering. Temporary fillings must be placed securely with proper thickness to resist dislodgement. Permanent restorations should be fitted as soon as possible, especially in teeth with large access cavities. Coronal leakage is one of the leading causes of postoperative microbial irritation and can be prevented with proper sealing and restoration planning.

Finally, prevention is strengthened by continuous evaluation during treatment. Clinicians must remain alert for anatomical complexities such as additional canals, isthmuses, or severe curvatures. Missed anatomy is one of the most common causes of postoperative complications and often results from rushed treatment or inadequate visualization. Using magnification, illumination, and CBCT imaging when indicated improves accuracy and reduces the chances of leaving untreated spaces that later become sources of irritation.

Together, this evidence based strategies offer a comprehensive approach to minimizing postoperative pain and swelling. They emphasize that prevention is not a single action but a chain of deliberate clinical decisions grounded in scientific understanding and careful execution. When applied consistently, these strategies enhance patient comfort, reduce complications, and improve the predictability of endodontic outcomes.

5.1 Preventive Value of Access Cavity Design and Canal Location

Access cavity design is one of the earliest procedural decisions that influence the outcome of root canal therapy, yet its role in preventing postoperative pain is often underestimated. A well designed access cavity provides straight line entry to the canals, reduces unnecessary dentin removal, and minimizes procedural errors that can irritate periapical tissues. In contrast, inadequate access can lead to instrument binding, canal transportation, missed anatomy, and inefficient irrigation, all of which increase the risk of postoperative inflammation.

When clinicians create a conservative but sufficiently open access cavity, instruments glide more smoothly within the canals. This reduces frictional heat and stress on the canal walls, lowering the risk of microcracks that can sensitize the periodontal ligament. Efficient access also prevents excessive force during glide path preparation and shaping, which helps minimize extrusion of debris into the periapical region. Without proper access, clinicians may unintentionally direct instruments toward the canal walls, increasing the likelihood of ledging or apical transportation, both of which irritate tissues and cause postoperative pain.

Another important preventive aspect of access cavity design involves accurate canal location. Missed canals are among the leading sources of post obturation complications. When untreated areas of pulp or microbial biofilm remain within the tooth, they continue to release toxins and inflammatory mediators long after obturation. These irritants diffuse toward the apex and provoke chronic or intermittent postoperative symptoms. Proper access cavity design facilitates identification of anatomical landmarks, enabling clinicians to locate additional canals such as MB2 in maxillary molars or lingual canals in mandibular incisors. Magnification and enhanced illumination further improve visibility and reduce the chance of missed anatomy.

Additionally, access cavities that provide optimal visibility allow clinicians to irrigate effectively since irrigants can reach the full length of the canal without obstruction. Restricted access often forces irrigants through narrow pathways with increased apical pressure, which significantly raises the risk of extrusion. By ensuring that irrigants flow freely through a well-shaped cavity, clinicians promote effective contact with canal walls while maintaining safety.

Overall, access cavity preparation is not merely a mechanical step but a preventive measure that influences every subsequent aspect of treatment. When clinicians understand the relationship between access design, instrument control, irrigation efficacy, and anatomical accuracy, they build a foundation that significantly reduces the likelihood of postoperative pain and swelling.

5.2 Role of Final Irrigation Protocols and Canal Disinfection in Preventing Persistent Symptoms

Final irrigation represents a critical phase of endodontic therapy that directly contributes to reducing postoperative complications. While instrumentation removes the bulk of infected tissue and debris, a significant percentage of microbial activity persists within untouched areas of the canal system. These regions include fins, isthmuses, apical deltas, and lateral canals where instruments cannot reach. Final irrigation protocols enhance disinfection by penetrating these areas, dissolving organic remnants, neutralizing endotoxins, and preparing the canal for obturation.

One of the most important aspects of final irrigation is the sequence of irrigants. Sodium hypochlorite remains the primary agent due to its ability to dissolve necrotic tissue and disrupt bacterial biofilms. When used in combination with EDTA, which removes the smear layer and exposes dentinal tubules, sodium hypochlorite becomes significantly more effective. The removal of the smear layer during final irrigation allows disinfecting agents to reach deeper into canal walls and eliminate bacteria that would otherwise contribute to postoperative irritation.

Activation methods greatly enhance the efficacy of final irrigation. Ultrasonic activation creates acoustic streaming and cavitation that disrupt biofilms and encourage irrigant movement into complex anatomical areas. Sonic activation and mechanical agitation using special devices also improve fluid penetration. These techniques increase the surface contact of irrigants without increasing apical pressure, which helps maintain safety while improving disinfection. The result is a cleaner canal system that is less likely to provoke inflammatory reactions after obturation.

The timing of irrigant activation is also relevant. Activating irrigants after shaping but before obturation ensures that debris generated during preparation is fully removed. If remnants of dentin or pulp tissue remain, they may undergo microbial degradation and release toxins that stimulate postoperative inflammation. A thorough final rinse with sodium hypochlorite followed by EDTA and a cleansing rinse with sterile saline or chlorhexidine reduces this risk.

Another preventive factor involves controlling canal dryness. Proper drying prevents sealer dilution and incomplete polymerization. When sealer does not set correctly, chemical components may leach into periapical tissues and cause irritation. Paper points should be used until dry, and clinicians must avoid excessive drying that may fracture fragile canal walls or desiccate dentin.

Equally important is ensuring that irrigants do not extrude beyond the apex during the final stages of disinfection. Apical extrusion during final irrigation is particularly dangerous because it exposes periapical tissues to concentrated chemical agents at the very end of treatment, when tissues are already sensitized from instrumentation. Using side venting needles, maintaining adequate distance from the apex, and applying slow, controlled irrigation prevents this complication.

The effectiveness of final irrigation has a direct influence on the incidence of persistent postoperative symptoms. When microbial load is reduced to its lowest possible level, the inflammatory response in the periapical region becomes more stable and predictable. This allows tissues to begin healing immediately after obturation, resulting in fewer complications and faster resolution of discomfort.

CHAPTER 6

Pharmacological Management of Post Obturation Pain and Swelling

Pharmacological management is a critical component of endodontic care because it directly addresses the inflammatory and nociceptive processes that shape the patient's postoperative experience. Although mechanical and microbial factors determine the origin of pain, medications influence how the body responds to these triggers. A well informed pharmacologic strategy reduces discomfort, supports tissue healing, and minimizes the likelihood of complications. This chapter explores the evidence based medications used to manage post obturation pain and swelling, highlighting their mechanisms, indications, limitations, and role in comprehensive patient care.

Pain following endodontic therapy arises primarily from inflammation in periapical tissues. When instrumentation, irrigation, or microbial remnants irritate these tissues, the body initiates a cascade of inflammatory signals involving prostaglandins, bradykinin, histamine, and cytokines. These mediators sensitize nociceptors and increase vascular permeability, resulting in pain and edema. Pharmacologic agents target different parts of this cascade, either reducing inflammation or modulating pain pathways to improve patient comfort.

Non steroidal anti-inflammatory drugs remain the first line medications for managing post obturation discomfort. NSAIDs such as ibuprofen, naproxen, and diclofenac inhibit cyclooxygenase enzymes, which are responsible for prostaglandin synthesis. By reducing prostaglandins, these medications diminish both inflammation and nociceptor sensitization. Numerous clinical trials demonstrate that NSAIDs offer superior pain relief compared to acetaminophen for inflammatory dental pain. They are particularly beneficial during the first twenty four to forty eight hours after treatment, when inflammatory activity peaks. However, NSAIDs must be prescribed with caution in patients with gastrointestinal disease, kidney impairment, cardiovascular conditions, or a history of allergy to these medications.

Acetaminophen plays an important complementary role in analgesia. While it does not possess strong peripheral anti inflammatory effects, it modulates pain perception centrally and enhances the effectiveness of NSAIDs when used in combination. Evidence shows that alternating or combining acetaminophen with ibuprofen produces stronger analgesia than either drug alone. This combination is especially useful in patients who experience moderate to severe discomfort but do not exhibit significant swelling or inflammation. Acetaminophen remains safe for patients who cannot tolerate NSAIDs, provided they do not exceed recommended dosage limits to avoid hepatic toxicity.

For cases involving significant inflammation or early flare ups, corticosteroids may be indicated. Corticosteroids reduce inflammation by inhibiting phospholipase A2, an enzyme responsible for initiating the arachidonic acid pathway that leads to prostaglandin and leukotriene production. This suppression reduces swelling and limits tissue sensitivity. Systemic corticosteroids such as prednisone or dexamethasone have been shown to decrease both the intensity and duration of postoperative pain when administered shortly after treatment. Some clinicians also use intracanal corticosteroid medicaments in select cases, although systemic administration remains more predictable. Corticosteroids must be used carefully in patients with diabetes, hypertension, immune compromise, or gastrointestinal ulcers.

Antibiotics are often misunderstood in the context of postoperative pain. Evidence clearly shows that antibiotics do not reduce pain following endodontic therapy unless there is an active spreading infection with systemic involvement. Pain alone, without swelling, fever, or cellulitis, is not an indication for antibiotic therapy. Overuse of antibiotics contributes to resistance and exposes patients to unnecessary side effects. Appropriate indications for antibiotics include facial swelling, lymphadenitis, trismus, fever, or signs of systemic spread. When indicated, common regimens include amoxicillin or, in the case of penicillin allergy, clindamycin. For severe infections, amoxicillin combined with clavulanic acid may be necessary.

Another important pharmacological consideration is the use of local anesthetic agents during treatment. Long acting anesthetics such as bupivacaine offer extended postoperative pain control, especially in patients undergoing procedures associated with high levels of tissue manipulation. By providing prolonged numbness, these agents reduce the immediate inflammatory response and give patients greater comfort during the early healing period. While the anesthetic effect itself is temporary, the reduction in early pain contributes to lower overall postoperative discomfort.

Adjunctive medications also have value in specific circumstances. Muscle relaxants may be beneficial when postoperative pain is exacerbated by muscular tension, particularly in patients who clench or grind during sleep. These habits can intensify periodontal ligament inflammation and prolong recovery. Antihistamines and gastric protectants may support patients who require high dose NSAID therapy but are at risk for gastrointestinal irritation.

The pharmacologic approach must always consider the patient's overall health status and medication history. Patients with chronic inflammatory diseases may exhibit heightened postoperative pain because of altered immune regulation. Those taking anticoagulants may require modified pain management plans to avoid interactions. Pregnant or breastfeeding patients require medications with established safety records. Understanding these variables ensures that pharmacologic therapy is effective, safe, and tailored to the individual.

Effective pharmacologic management also depends on clear communication. Patients must understand when and how to take medications, what symptoms require attention, and what level of discomfort is normal. Misuse or inconsistent dosing reduces medication effectiveness and may lead patients to believe their pain is a sign of treatment failure. When clinicians educate patients thoroughly, pharmacologic interventions become more predictable and reassuring.

Pharmacologic management also extends beyond treating pain. Proper use of medications helps stabilize the inflammatory response, allowing tissues to heal more efficiently. When swelling is controlled early, vascular congestion decreases, and lymphatic drainage improves. When pain is moderated, patients experience less anxiety and muscle tension, both of which influence the perception of discomfort. Pharmacologic therapy, therefore, contributes not only to immediate relief but also to the long term success of endodontic healing.

Taken together, the pharmacological tools available to clinicians provide powerful means of supporting patients through the postoperative period. By choosing the appropriate combination of NSAIDs, acetaminophen, corticosteroids, and adjunctive medications, and by reserving antibiotics for true infections, clinicians can significantly reduce the burden of post obturation symptoms. Pharmacologic therapy complements mechanical precision and microbial control, forming an essential part of a comprehensive strategy to minimize postoperative complications and enhance patient satisfaction.

6.1 Timing and Dosing Strategies for Optimal Pharmacologic Control

The effectiveness of pharmacologic management in endodontics is influenced not only by the type of medication prescribed but also by the timing and dosing schedule. Pain perception is closely tied to the inflammatory cycle, which evolves rapidly during the first twenty four to seventy two hours after obturation. Clinicians who understand these temporal dynamics are better equipped to tailor medication regimens that prevent the escalation of inflammation rather than simply reacting to it.

Research demonstrates that preemptive analgesia reduces postoperative discomfort by interrupting the inflammatory cascade before it becomes established. Administering NSAIDs shortly before treatment decreases the production of prostaglandins that are stimulated by instrumentation and irrigation. When prostaglandin synthesis is controlled early, nociceptors are less sensitized, which leads to lower pain intensity during the early postoperative period. This strategy is particularly beneficial for patients with symptomatic apical periodontitis, where preexisting inflammation amplifies postoperative responses.

Postoperative dosing is equally important. NSAIDs should be administered on a scheduled basis rather than waiting for pain to escalate. Consistent dosing maintains inhibition of cyclooxygenase enzymes and prevents breakthrough pain that becomes more difficult to manage once it is established. For example, ibuprofen taken every six to eight hours provides better pain control than taking it only when symptoms worsen. Combining acetaminophen with scheduled NSAID use enhances analgesic coverage by utilizing different mechanisms of action.

Corticosteroids benefit greatly from early administration. A single dose given immediately after treatment has been shown to significantly reduce swelling and pain during the first forty eight hours. The timing is critical because corticosteroids act upstream in the inflammatory pathway, preventing the formation of both prostaglandins and leukotrienes. If administered too late, their impact on swelling and nociceptor sensitization is reduced.

Adjusting dose intensity is also necessary for individual patients. Those experiencing severe inflammation or undergoing procedures involving significant manipulation, such as retreatment or complex molar therapy, may require higher initial doses. However, clinical judgment must balance analgesic effectiveness with safety considerations based on age, systemic diseases, and concurrent medications.

Together, precise timing and individualized dosing strategies form a sophisticated component of pharmacologic prevention. They ensure that medications work in harmony with biological processes rather than against them, producing smoother recoveries and fewer complications.

6.2 Patient Specific Considerations and Risk Factors in Pharmacologic Planning

Effective pharmacologic management must account for the unique characteristics and health status of each patient. While medications such as NSAIDs, acetaminophen, and corticosteroids are widely used, their safety and effectiveness vary according to systemic conditions, allergies, organ function, and physiological responses. Failure to tailor pharmacologic strategies to individual risk factors increases the likelihood of adverse reactions and reduces therapeutic benefit.

Patients with cardiovascular disease, kidney impairment, or gastrointestinal disorders require modified NSAID therapy. NSAIDs may increase blood pressure, reduce renal perfusion, or irritate the gastric mucosa. These risks necessitate lower dosages, shorter treatment durations, or alternative analgesics. Acetaminophen becomes the preferred primary analgesic for many of these patients because it lacks peripheral anti inflammatory effects that burden the kidneys or gastrointestinal system. Clinicians must also account for maximum daily doses to avoid hepatotoxicity, especially in patients who consume alcohol regularly or take medications metabolized by the liver.

Patients with diabetes or immune compromise may experience stronger postoperative inflammatory responses due to altered immune system regulation. These individuals may benefit from cautious corticosteroid use, but their systemic conditions must be monitored closely because steroids can influence glucose levels and immune function. For diabetic patients, a short course of low dose corticosteroids may offer substantial symptom relief without significantly elevating risk, but only when the clinician communicates clearly with the patient regarding glucose monitoring.

Anxiety prone patients represent another group requiring tailored pharmacologic planning. Anxiety amplifies pain perception and can cause muscle tension that worsens postoperative discomfort. These patients benefit not only from effective analgesics but also from clear communication, reassurance, and when appropriate, adjunctive medications such as mild muscle relaxants. Reducing anxiety enhances the effectiveness of pharmacologic pain control by lowering the patient's overall pain sensitivity.

A history of allergies must also be integrated into pharmacologic decisions. Patients allergic to aspirin or other NSAIDs may require acetaminophen based regimens. Those allergic to penicillin require alternative antibiotics such as clindamycin when infection is present. Patients with multiple drug allergies may need more complex management involving careful selection of safe and effective substitutes.

Age is an additional factor. Elderly patients often have reduced renal function or take multiple medications that interact with common analgesics. Pediatric patients require weight based dosing and medications with favorable safety profiles. Pregnant and breastfeeding patients require medications with established safety histories, avoiding drugs that cross the placenta or are excreted in breast milk at high concentrations.

In all cases, clinicians must conduct a thorough medical history review and document medication use, allergies, and systemic risks before prescribing pharmacologic agents. When tailored appropriately, medication regimens become safer, more predictable, and more effective at managing post obturation pain and swelling.

CHAPTER 7

Diagnostic Reasoning for Persistent Post Obturation Symptoms and Clinical Decision Making

Persistent postoperative pain or swelling after root canal therapy presents one of the most difficult challenges for clinicians, not because these symptoms are rare but because they can arise from multiple biological and mechanical factors that interact in complex ways. The success of endodontic treatment depends not only on technical skill but also on the clinician's ability to evaluate symptoms accurately, interpret clinical signs, select appropriate interventions, and distinguish true complications from normal healing responses. Chapter 7 focuses on the structured clinical reasoning required to diagnose persistent symptoms and make decisions that prevent escalation, avoid unnecessary retreatment, and ensure patient safety.

Accurate diagnosis begins with a deliberate and methodical approach. The clinician must revisit the patient's symptom history, noting changes in intensity, frequency, and character since obturation. Persistent discomfort that remains stable or gradually improves usually reflects normal tissue healing. In contrast, symptoms that intensify over several days suggest underlying irritation or microbial persistence that requires further investigation. Sharp pain on biting may reflect occlusal overload or a cracked cusp, while continuous throbbing accompanied by a feeling of pressure often suggests developing inflammation around the apex. These distinctions, though subtle, influence treatment decisions significantly.

Clinical examination provides additional clarity. Palpation over the periapical tissues reveals whether inflammation is localized or spreading. Percussion testing indicates the sensitivity of periodontal tissues and helps differentiate between normal healing and an acute inflammatory process. The presence of swelling, whether diffuse or localized, signals the progression of inflammation beyond the canal and into adjacent tissues. Warmth, fluctuation, and vestibular fullness must be documented carefully because their presence determines whether conservative management is appropriate or whether drainage and pharmacologic intervention are needed.

A thorough assessment always includes occlusal evaluation. Minor occlusal discrepancies can magnify postoperative symptoms, particularly in teeth recovering from recent instrumentation. When a tooth is placed under excessive bite force, the periodontal ligament becomes overstressed, leading to heightened inflammation and prolonged pain. In such cases, simple occlusal adjustment may resolve the symptoms without additional intervention. This diagnostic insight prevents unnecessary retreatment and reinforces the importance of systematic evaluation.

Radiographic imaging plays a central role in decision making. A postoperative periapical radiograph allows the clinician to evaluate obturation quality, working length, density, and the presence of voids or overextensions. Underfilling or uninstrumented areas may harbor microbial biofilms that continually irritate apical tissues. Overextended sealer or gutta percha may provoke foreign body reactions. In cases where radiographs are inconclusive, cone beam computed tomography provides a more detailed view of anatomical complexity, hidden canals, fractures, resorption, or periapical pathology. CBCT imaging is especially valuable when persistent symptoms cannot be explained by clinical examination alone.

Understanding the timeline of symptom development is another key diagnostic element. Mild to moderate sensitivity immediately after treatment is expected. Swelling and severe pain within the first twenty four hours may indicate debris extrusion or aggressive inflammation. Symptoms that develop several days later suggest a delayed immune response or microbial leakage. Pain that appears weeks after treatment often indicates coronal infiltration, missed anatomy, or microleakage through a failing restoration. These temporal patterns allow clinicians to predict causes with greater accuracy and choose interventions that match the biological state of the tissues.

Differential diagnosis is essential in cases of persistent symptoms. Post obturation pain may be confused with periodontal disease, cracked tooth syndrome, temporomandibular joint dysfunction, sinusitis, or referred pain from musculature. Each of these conditions presents with pain that may mimic apical pathology. A tooth with a vertical root fracture may show early relief after treatment followed by recurrent pain and swelling. A tooth affected by sinus pressure may display tenderness on percussion but not respond predictably to endodontic treatment. Without careful differential diagnosis, unnecessary retreatment may occur, offering no benefit and introducing additional risk.

Decision making must also incorporate microbial considerations. Persistent symptoms may indicate the survival of bacteria within lateral canals, isthmuses, or uninstrumented segments of the canal system. Some microorganisms possess virulence factors that stimulate strong inflammatory responses even when present in small numbers. When microbial persistence is suspected, retreatment becomes an evidence based decision. Removing existing obturation material, reopening the canal, and applying enhanced irrigation protocols often provide rapid symptom relief. At other times, when persistent infection is located beyond the apex or within inaccessible anatomical regions, surgical intervention may be the preferred approach.

Non microbial causes require different strategies. If the discomfort results from occlusal overload, correcting the bite resolves inflammation quickly. If chemical irritation from extruded sealer is responsible, conservative management with monitoring and anti inflammatory medication is appropriate, as many cases improve spontaneously. If swelling is caused by pressure buildup within periapical tissues, drainage may offer immediate relief and prevent progression to abscess formation. These clinical decisions underscore the importance of interpreting symptoms within the broader biological context rather than reflexively choosing invasive procedures.

Patient communication is an integral part of diagnostic reasoning. Patients may interpret persistent discomfort as evidence of treatment failure, which increases anxiety and amplifies pain perception. When clinicians explain the healing process clearly, describe expected symptoms, and outline next steps based on diagnostic findings, patients become more confident and cooperative. Psychological reassurance reduces sympathetic nervous activation and supports faster recovery.

Another essential part of decision making involves understanding the patient's medical history. Systemic conditions such as diabetes, autoimmune disorders, or vascular disease influence healing capacity and inflammatory responses. Patients with exaggerated inflammatory tendencies may show prolonged postoperative discomfort despite flawless treatment. Recognizing these individual differences prevents misinterpretation of normal biological variation as pathology.

Ultimately, the clinician's goal in evaluating persistent post obturation symptoms is to determine whether the condition is improving, stable, or deteriorating. Improvement indicates that the body is healing and that supportive care may be all that is needed. Stability without improvement requires closer monitoring and possibly pharmacologic intervention. Deterioration demands immediate action, whether through occlusal adjustment, drainage, antibiotics in selective cases, or retreatment. By following a structured diagnostic process that incorporates history, examination, imaging, differential diagnosis, microbiology, and patient factors, clinicians can select appropriate interventions with confidence.

In summary, effective clinical decision making for persistent postoperative symptoms requires more than technical expertise. It demands thoughtful interpretation of biological signals, an understanding of tissue responses, and a disciplined commitment to evidence based reasoning. When these components are applied consistently, clinicians are able to protect patients from unnecessary discomfort, avoid overtreatment, and ensure long term treatment success.

7.1 Integrating Pain Quality and Pattern Recognition into Diagnostic Interpretation

One of the most powerful yet often underutilized diagnostic tools in endodontics is the careful analysis of pain characteristics. Pain quality, intensity, rhythm, and triggers provide insight into the biological processes occurring within the periapical region. Recognizing these patterns allows clinicians to distinguish between normal healing and pathological changes that require intervention.

Sharp, localized pain during chewing typically signals periodontal ligament inflammation or occlusal overload. In these cases, the pain originates from mechanical stress rather than infection, and occlusal adjustment may offer immediate relief. Conversely, continuous throbbing or pulsation often reflects vascular congestion within the periapical tissues. These symptoms correlate with increased interstitial pressure caused by inflammatory exudate and require anti-inflammatory strategies or drainage depending on severity.

A dull, lingering ache that persists regardless of chewing may indicate low grade microbial irritation within untreated anatomical spaces. This pattern often appears when a canal was missed or when biofilms persist in areas inaccessible to instruments. Pain that worsens at night may reflect vascular changes associated with lying down, which increases blood flow to the head and intensifies inflammatory pressure.

Identifying these distinctions is essential for accurate diagnosis. Pain triggered by thermal changes after obturation may signal residual sensitivity from instrumentation but could also suggest coronal leakage or microcracks. Pain described as a sudden shock or electric sensation can indicate a cracked tooth rather than an endodontic failure. Recognizing the unique signatures of different pain categories helps clinicians avoid misinterpreting symptoms and choosing inappropriate treatments.

By teaching clinicians to interpret pain as a diagnostic language, this approach enhances accuracy and confidence in decision making and reduces unnecessary interventions.

7.2 Differentiating Radiographic Healing Patterns from Pathological Changes

Radiographs remain one of the most valuable diagnostic tools in endodontics, yet their interpretation requires more than identifying voids, overfills, or lesions. Subtle differences in radiographic healing patterns can reveal whether a postoperative symptom is part of normal recovery or a sign of persistent pathology.

Early postoperative radiographs often show slight widening of the periodontal ligament space, which reflects acute inflammation rather than treatment failure. This widening may persist for several weeks without indicating a complication. In contrast, progressive widening over time suggests sustained irritation or microbial persistence, particularly if accompanied by worsening symptoms.

Radiolucencies around the apex require careful interpretation. A stable radiolucency after treatment is common when preoperative lesions were present, as bone remodeling requires months to become radiographically evident. A decrease in radiolucency over time indicates healing, even if the patient experiences intermittent tenderness. Increasing radiolucency, however, signals continued pathology and may require retreatment.

Overextended materials appear radiopaque beyond the apex, but not all overextensions cause pain. Small amounts of sealer extrusion often become encapsulated by connective tissue and do not necessitate intervention. However, persistent pain combined with radiographic extrusion may indicate a foreign body reaction, especially if symptoms localize to the affected root.

Cone beam computed tomography clarifies ambiguous findings by providing three dimensional visualization of canal anatomy, fractures, uninstrumented segments, and periapical structures. CBCT imaging is particularly helpful in teeth with persistent symptoms but unclear periapical changes on conventional radiographs.

By integrating radiographic interpretation with clinical findings, clinicians can differentiate between healing, stagnation, and deterioration, thus selecting appropriate next steps with greater precision.

7.3 Clinical Decision Pathways for Managing Persistent Post Obturation Symptoms

Effective management of persistent postoperative symptoms requires structured decision pathways that guide clinicians from assessment to intervention. These pathways reduce uncertainty and ensure that diagnostic information is translated into action logically and consistently.

The first decision point is determining whether symptoms indicate normal healing or pathology. If symptoms are decreasing and there is no swelling, fever, or radiographic progression, conservative management with analgesics and monitoring is appropriate. The clinician should reassure the patient and schedule follow up evaluation.

The second pathway focuses on occlusal factors. If pain occurs primarily during chewing or biting, occlusal adjustment should be considered before more invasive interventions. Many cases resolve once excessive loading is eliminated, especially in posterior teeth.

The third pathway examines microbial factors. If symptoms persist beyond one to two weeks without improvement, or if radiographs suggest underfilling or missed anatomy, microbial involvement is likely. In these cases, retreatment becomes the next logical step. Removing obturation material, reinstrumenting canals, and applying enhanced irrigation often result in rapid symptom relief.

The fourth pathway addresses acute flare ups. If swelling, fever, or rapidly escalating pain is present, immediate management is required. This may include drainage, anti-inflammatory medication, and, when appropriate, antibiotics. Once acute inflammation subsides, the clinician reassesses and determines whether retreatment or surgical intervention is necessary.

The fifth pathway involves evaluating fractures or structural compromise. If clinical tests or CBCT imaging indicate a cracked root or vertical fracture, extraction or prosthetic planning may be required. Recognizing this early prevents unnecessary retreatment and prolonged discomfort.

By following structured pathways rather than relying solely on intuition, clinicians enhance diagnostic accuracy, improve patient outcomes, and avoid unnecessary or ineffective procedures.

Case Study 1: Persistent Pain After Molar Root Canal Therapy Misdiagnosis Avoided Through Structured Clinical Reasoning

A 41 year old civil engineer presented to the clinic eight days after root canal therapy on the lower left first molar. The procedure had been performed elsewhere, and the patient arrived visibly anxious, reporting that the pain had not resolved as he expected.

He described the discomfort as a constant dull ache with occasional sharp sensations when chewing. He had been taking over the counter analgesics with minimal relief. The patient believed the treatment had failed and requested extraction.

The clinician began with a thorough symptom history. The patient reported that pain immediately after treatment was mild, but by the third day, the discomfort increased. He denied any swelling, fever, or night pain. This temporal pattern suggested the possibility of occlusal overload or persistent inflammation rather than a spreading infection. The patient also mentioned that he avoided chewing on the affected side, yet light contact during swallowing triggered discomfort. This detail raised suspicion of periodontal ligament irritation.

Clinical examination was performed next. Extraoral tissues were normal, with no swelling or asymmetry. Intraoral inspection revealed a tooth with an intact temporary filling and no signs of drainage. Palpation over the buccal and lingual aspects produced mild tenderness but no fluctuance. Percussion elicited moderate discomfort, indicating ongoing periodontal inflammation. However, the most revealing test was bite evaluation using a bite stick. When pressure was applied to the mesiobuccal cusp, the patient experienced significant sharp pain, while other cusps caused minimal discomfort.

This pain pattern often indicates occlusal overload rather than an endodontic failure. To verify, the clinician assessed the occlusion using articulating paper. The treated molar displayed a heavy premature contact in maximum intercuspation, created inadvertently during the earlier restoration. This high contact transferred excessive forces to the inflamed periodontal ligament, perpetuating the patient's discomfort.

Radiographic evaluation provided further clarity. A periapical radiograph showed well condensed obturation, proper working length, and no voids. The periodontal ligament space was slightly widened but stable, consistent with postoperative inflammation. There was no evidence of missed canals or progressive radiolucency.

Based on the structured diagnostic process, the clinician concluded that the pain was caused primarily by occlusal trauma rather than persistent infection or endodontic failure. Occlusal adjustment was performed by reducing the high contact and balancing the bite. The patient was prescribed an anti inflammatory medication and instructed to monitor symptoms over the next forty eight hours.

Within two days, the patient reported dramatic improvement, and by the one week follow up, all symptoms had resolved. This case illustrates how structured assessment prevents unnecessary retreatment or extraction. Without careful evaluation, the patient's request for removal of the tooth might have been accepted, leading to loss of a tooth with a perfectly adequate root canal treatment.

Case Study 2: Swelling and Severe Pain Two Weeks After Treatment Discovery of Missed Anatomy Through Diagnostic Pathways

A 56 year old nurse arrived complaining of increasing pain and swelling around the upper right first molar. She had undergone root canal therapy two weeks earlier for a chronic periapical lesion. Initially, her symptoms improved, but ten days after treatment, she noticed mild discomfort that progressed into severe throbbing pain. By the time she presented, the swelling had extended into the buccal vestibule, though she remained afebrile.

The clinician gathered a detailed history. The patient explained that she felt normal for the first week, then began experiencing episodes of pressure that worsened during chewing. The delayed onset of symptoms suggested microbial persistence rather than chemical or mechanical irritation. The pain was described as rhythmic and pulsating, which often reflects inflammation driven by bacterial byproducts within the canal or periapical tissues.

Intraoral examination revealed localized swelling in the buccal vestibule of the maxillary molar region. The tissue was firm and warm but not yet fluctuant. Percussion produced sharp pain, especially over the mesiobuccal root. Palpation intensified discomfort, and biting pressure caused severe sensitivity. These findings suggested active inflammatory exacerbation rather than a simple healing reaction.

A periapical radiograph was taken and reviewed carefully. The obturation appeared adequate in two canals, but the mesiobuccal root displayed an obturation pattern consistent with a single canal filling. The clinician considered anatomical expectations. Maxillary first molars frequently contain two mesiobuccal canals, and failure to locate and treat the second canal is one of the most common causes of persistent symptoms.

To confirm the suspicion, cone beam computed tomography was ordered. The scan revealed a clearly identifiable untreated MB2 canal with a separate orifice and apical exit. The canal displayed radiographic evidence of debris and remnants of necrotic tissue. The surrounding periapical region showed increased radiolucency compared to the immediate postoperative radiograph, indicating progression of microbial activity.

Given the clinical findings and CBCT evidence, the clinician diagnosed a postoperative flare up caused by missed anatomy. Immediate management included relieving occlusal forces, prescribing NSAIDs for inflammation, and initiating antibiotics due to the presence of swelling and risk of space infection. After initial stabilization, formal retreatment was scheduled.

During retreatment, the mesiobuccal access was refined using magnification. The MB2 canal was located, cleaned, and shaped.

Irrigation was enhanced using ultrasonic activation to penetrate the complex anatomy. Calcium hydroxide was placed as an intracanal medicament to neutralize bacterial toxins and reduce inflammation. The patient reported improvement within forty eight hours, and swelling resolved by day three.

One week later, the canal system was obturated correctly. At the six week follow up, the patient reported complete resolution of symptoms, and radiographic evaluation indicated early signs of periapical healing.

This case underscores the importance of structured diagnostic pathways, proper imaging, and an understanding of anatomical variability. Without CBCT evaluation and methodical reasoning, the clinician might have misattributed the symptoms to normal postoperative sensitivity, delaying appropriate intervention and risking further complications.

CHAPTER 8

Treatment Protocols for Persistent Post Obturation Pain and Swelling

Persistent pain or swelling after root canal therapy represents a clinical situation that demands thoughtful, evidence based intervention. While most postoperative symptoms resolve within a few days, a subset of cases continues to present discomfort or develops new complications that signal the need for active treatment. The goal of this chapter is to provide a comprehensive framework for managing these situations with accuracy and confidence. Successful intervention relies on identifying the biological source of irritation, selecting the least invasive treatment capable of resolving the issue, and preventing escalation into chronic pathology or systemic involvement.

The first step in formulating an appropriate treatment strategy is differentiating between conditions that require conservative management and those that necessitate procedural intervention. Persistent mild sensitivity without swelling is often the result of lingering periodontal ligament inflammation. In such cases, anti-inflammatory medications, occlusal adjustment, and reassurance form the basis of care. Patients frequently respond within forty eight to seventy two hours once mechanical stress is reduced and inflammation stabilizes. This conservative approach avoids unnecessary retreatment while supporting the natural healing process.

When symptoms suggest microbial persistence rather than mechanical irritation, intervention becomes more complex. Microorganisms may remain within lateral canals, isthmuses, or uninstrumented segments of the root canal system. In these cases, the inflammatory response continues despite an apparently well completed obturation. Retreatment becomes the preferred protocol because it allows the clinician to reaccess the canal system, remove filling materials, and apply enhanced disinfection strategies. Evidence consistently shows that retreatment is highly effective when persistent pain originates from untreated or insufficiently disinfected anatomy. During retreatment, clinicians should refine the access cavity, search for additional canals, use magnification, and incorporate activated irrigation to improve microbial control.

Some cases of persistent discomfort arise from extruded filling materials, particularly when sealer or gutta percha extends significantly beyond the apex. While many extrusions become encapsulated and asymptomatic, others provoke chronic inflammation or foreign body reactions. Treatment depends on the severity of symptoms. When discomfort is mild, observation and pharmacologic support may be appropriate. If symptoms worsen or persist for several months, surgical intervention such as apicoectomy allows removal of extruded material and curettage of inflamed periapical tissues. This approach is minimally invasive but highly effective when conservative measures fail.

Acute flare ups require immediate clinical management. These episodes occur when microbial byproducts, debris, or pressure accumulate in the periapical region. Patients present with severe pain, swelling, and in some cases, limited mouth opening. The primary goal is rapid reduction of tissue pressure and inflammation. Drainage, either through the canal or by soft tissue incision, provides immediate relief by releasing accumulated exudate. Once drainage is achieved, intracanal medication such as calcium hydroxide reduces bacterial load and stabilizes the tissues. Pharmacologic support with NSAIDs and, when indicated, antibiotics is essential for controlling spreading inflammation. After stabilizing the acute condition, the clinician reassesses whether retreatment or completion of obturation is appropriate.

Microleakage represents another important cause of persistent postoperative symptoms. When a temporary restoration fails or a permanent restoration lacks adequate sealing, oral bacteria enter the canal system and stimulate recurrent inflammation. Treatment requires immediate replacement or repair of the coronal seal to prevent further contamination. In cases where infiltration has occurred for an extended period, retreatment may be required to eliminate newly introduced microorganisms. This underscores the importance of protecting the coronal access during every stage of treatment to prevent iatrogenic complications.

Vertical root fractures represent a more serious cause of persistent postoperative symptoms. These fractures often produce intermittent swelling, localized pain on biting, and narrow periodontal pockets. Diagnosis requires careful evaluation, often with cone beam computed tomography. Unfortunately, vertical root fractures cannot be repaired and typically require extraction. Recognizing the signs early prevents unnecessary retreatment and reduces the risk of chronic infection. Although extraction is an undesirable outcome, accurate diagnosis preserves surrounding tissues and enables timely planning for implants or prosthetic rehabilitation.

Surgical endodontic intervention is indicated when persistent symptoms originate from anatomical challenges or inaccessible microbial reservoirs. Apicoectomy with retrograde sealing allows the clinician to address periapical pathology directly, remove granulation tissue, and seal the apical anatomy from the root end. This approach is beneficial when the canal cannot be retreated due to obstructions, posts, fractures, or severe curvatures. Modern microsurgical techniques using ultrasonic retropreparation and bioceramic retroseal materials offer high success rates for cases previously considered untreatable.

Another important treatment protocol involves managing persistent neuropathic pain. In rare cases, postoperative pain persists even in the absence of inflammation or infection. This neuropathic pain may arise from sensitization of nerve fibers or central processing pathways. Treatment includes referral to a pain specialist, use of neuropathic medications such as gabapentin, and management strategies that focus on restoring normal sensory function. Recognizing neuropathic pain prevents unnecessary and ineffective dental retreatment.

Effective management of persistent complications also requires patient education. Clear explanation of the steps being taken and the reasoning behind them reduces anxiety, which itself can amplify pain perception. When patients understand the nature of their symptoms and the expected course of treatment, compliance improves and outcomes become more predictable.

Overall, treatment protocols for persistent post obturation complications require a delicate balance between conservative monitoring and timely intervention. Clinicians must recognize when symptoms reflect healing, when they signal microbial persistence, and when they indicate mechanical or anatomical challenges. By applying structured diagnostic reasoning and evidence based treatment strategies, clinicians can resolve complications efficiently, protect patient comfort, and ensure the long term success of endodontic therapy.

8.1 The Role of Intracanal Medicaments in Managing Persistent Inflammation

Intracanal medicaments play a central role in resolving persistent postoperative symptoms, particularly when discomfort is driven by microbial activity or residual toxins within the canal system. While chemo mechanical debridement remains the foundation of endodontic disinfection, medicaments provide sustained antimicrobial activity that continues long after instrumentation is complete. Calcium hydroxide remains the most extensively studied material for this purpose. Its high pH disrupts bacterial cell membranes, denatures proteins, and neutralizes endotoxins that can perpetuate inflammation even in the absence of viable microorganisms. When placed within the canal for seven to fourteen days, calcium hydroxide reduces bacterial loads to levels unattainable through mechanical cleaning alone. The medicament also promotes periapical healing by inhibiting osteoclastic activity and stimulating the formation of hard tissue barriers.

In cases with persistent swelling or pain that does not respond to initial retreatment, calcium hydroxide can be used as an extended therapeutic phase. It is particularly helpful in cases involving complex anatomy where complete cleaning is difficult. When persistent symptoms arise from anaerobic bacterial communities deep within canal irregularities, placing calcium hydroxide ensures a prolonged period of antimicrobial action and creates conditions unfavorable for microbial survival. Other medicaments, including chlorhexidine based formulations and bioactive gels, may serve as adjuncts in select situations, particularly when dealing with resistant species. The clinician must ensure that medicaments are properly sealed within the canal to prevent coronal leakage and maintain therapeutic concentration. By integrating intracanal medicaments into a structured treatment protocol, clinicians enhance the likelihood of symptom resolution and increase the long term success of retreatment procedures.

8.2 Surgical Decision Making for Complications Unresponsive to Conventional Treatment

When persistent pain or swelling fails to resolve after retreatment and medicament therapy, surgical endodontic intervention becomes an essential component of the treatment protocol. Surgical management allows direct access to the apical region, enabling removal of infected tissue, granulation tissue, or foreign bodies that cannot be reached through conventional canal treatment. Apicoectomy combined with retrograde sealing is the most common surgical approach. During this procedure, the clinician resects the apical portion of the root, curettes the periapical pathology, and prepares a retrograde cavity to seal the apical canal from the root end. Modern microsurgical techniques use magnification, ultrasonic instrumentation, and bioceramic materials that provide excellent sealing and biocompatibility, resulting in significantly higher success rates than older techniques.

Surgical intervention is especially useful when structural obstacles prevent traditional retreatment. Teeth with posts that cannot be removed safely, severely curved or calcified canals, or fractured instruments lodged deep within the root may not allow adequate conventional cleaning. In these situations, surgical access becomes the only predictable method for removing irritants and reestablishing apical health. Surgery is also indicated when periapical pathology persists despite meticulous retreatment, suggesting the presence of anatomical complexities or extra radicular infection. It is essential for clinicians to evaluate each case comprehensively, considering the patient's medical history, periodontal condition, anatomical variations, and restorative prognosis before choosing surgery. When performed under proper indications, endodontic surgery offers rapid symptom resolution and allows preservation of teeth that would otherwise be extracted.

CHAPTER 9

Advanced Clinical Assessment and Diagnostic Pathways for Post Obturation Pain and Swelling

Accurate assessment of postoperative pain and swelling remains one of the most critical responsibilities in endodontic practice, because the clinician's judgment determines whether a patient requires reassurance, conservative care, retreatment, or urgent intervention. Persistent symptoms may reflect normal healing, but they may also signal microbial persistence, mechanical irritation, inflammatory flare ups, or pathological changes in surrounding tissues. Chapter 9 deepens the clinician's interpretive skills by presenting advanced diagnostic strategies that integrate clinical examination, radiographic interpretation, symptom analysis, and an understanding of tissue biology.

The foundation of advanced diagnostic reasoning begins with the clinician's ability to distinguish between expected postoperative discomfort and symptoms that exceed the normal healing trajectory. Mild tenderness to percussion within the first few days is considered acceptable as the periodontal ligament recovers from instrumentation and apical exposure. However, pain that intensifies after forty eight to seventy two hours, or swelling that appears after an initial period of improvement, signals an underlying complication that must be investigated. These patterns provide the first clues that guide further diagnostic steps.

A detailed pain history is essential. The clinician must determine the exact onset, location, triggers, and progression of symptoms. Pain upon biting often reflects mechanical overload or microcracks, while spontaneous throbbing indicates vascular pressure within inflamed periapical tissues. Pain that radiates to neighboring teeth or structures suggests involvement of adjacent musculature or referred pain rather than endodontic failure. These distinctions are critical because pain patterns provide insight into the biological source of irritation. Without careful history taking, the clinician risks misdirecting the diagnostic process.

Clinical examination deepens this evaluative process. Palpation over the apices reveals whether inflammation is confined or spreading. When palpation is painful only directly over the affected tooth, the inflammation is usually localized. When palpation produces discomfort over a broader region or along the vestibule, it suggests more advanced tissue involvement. Percussion tests help quantify the severity of periodontal ligament inflammation, while gentle probing reveals whether periodontal pockets have deepened due to cracks or combined lesions. Thermal testing, although less commonly used after obturation, may offer additional diagnostic clues if the tooth responds abnormally.

Radiographic interpretation forms another central part of assessment. A postoperative radiograph provides a baseline for comparison. Clinicians must evaluate obturation length, density, voids, canal curvature, and evidence of untreated anatomy. If symptoms persist, additional radiographs taken at varying angulations may reveal hidden roots, missed canals, apical bifurcations, or subtle signs of overextension. Cone beam computed tomography expands this diagnostic capacity by providing three dimensional views that expose fractures, resorption, external inflammatory lesions, and the true shape of complex canal systems. CBCT is invaluable when conventional radiographs are inconclusive or when symptoms do not align with visible radiographic findings.

Beyond mechanical and microbial factors, advanced diagnosis requires evaluating the biological state of the tissues. Postoperative swelling can arise from microbial irritation, inflammatory mediators, or pressure imbalances within periapical spaces. Swelling that progresses rapidly indicates the presence of virulent microorganisms or expanding exudate that requires immediate management. Swelling that remains localized and nonfluctuant may reflect tissue inflammation rather than abscess formation. Distinguishing these presentations ensures that patients receive appropriate levels of care and helps clinicians avoid unnecessary incision or drainage procedures.

Coronal leakage is another important consideration in advanced assessment. Even minor defects in temporary or permanent restorations allow microorganisms to enter the canal system and stimulate recurrent symptoms. In such cases, the clinician must examine the integrity of the coronal seal, identify marginal breakdown, and determine whether contamination has progressed far enough to justify retreatment. Coronal leakage is often misdiagnosed as endodontic failure when, in reality, restoration repair would resolve the issue. A systematic evaluation of coronal structures prevents this error.

Occlusal evaluation is also essential. Even when a root canal procedure is technically flawless, excessive occlusal forces can inflame the periodontal ligament and prolong postoperative discomfort. Heavy biting contacts discovered through articulating paper or bite mapping often explain persistent symptoms. Adjusting the occlusion may provide immediate relief and restore normal function. This simple intervention highlights the importance of considering mechanical factors in the diagnostic process.

Another advanced element of assessment involves identifying non endodontic sources of pain. Temporomandibular joint disorders, myofascial pain, sinus inflammation, and neuralgia can all mimic endodontic symptoms. For example, maxillary posterior teeth often display tenderness caused by sinus pressure rather than periapical pathology. Similarly, referred pain from the masseter or temporalis muscle may lead patients to believe that a tooth is the source of discomfort. The clinician must be aware of these possibilities and use differential testing to exclude non dental causes.

Medical history evaluation forms the final component of advanced diagnostic assessment. Conditions such as diabetes, immune disorders, and vascular deficiencies alter healing capacity and inflammation responses. Patients with heightened inflammatory tendencies may experience prolonged discomfort despite excellent treatment outcomes. Understanding individual biological variability helps clinicians differentiate between pathological symptoms and normal but extended healing.

Once all diagnostic data has been gathered, the clinician must synthesize the information to determine the appropriate pathway of care. If symptoms reflect normal healing, reassurance and supportive management are indicated. If microbial persistence is suspected, retreatment becomes the logical choice. If structural damage or fractures are identified, extraction or surgical intervention may be required. The clinician's ability to integrate findings from multiple diagnostic sources ensures that the chosen treatment pathway aligns with the true underlying cause of symptoms.

In summary, advanced clinical assessment requires a comprehensive understanding of biological healing patterns, symptom expression, radiographic interpretation, and differential diagnosis. It demands disciplined reasoning that avoids assumptions and relies instead on systematic evaluation. By refining these diagnostic skills, clinicians enhance treatment outcomes, prevent unnecessary interventions, and ensure that patients receive accurate and timely care. Chapter 9 provides the foundation for this evaluative approach and prepares clinicians for the final management and prevention strategies explored in the concluding section of this work.

9.1 Integrating Clinical Imaging with Biological Interpretation for Accurate Diagnosis

Advanced diagnosis in endodontics requires more than taking radiographs. It demands an interpretive mindset that connects imaging findings with biological processes occurring within the periapical region. A radiograph provides a static view, but the clinician must decode it in the context of tissue dynamics, healing timelines, and microbial behavior. For example, a slight increase in radiolucency after obturation may not signal treatment failure. Instead, it may reflect transient bone resorption triggered by an inflammatory flare that is already beginning to resolve. Without understanding the biological meaning of this process, the clinician might assume that disease progression is occurring and choose an unnecessary retreatment.

Cone beam computed tomography enhances diagnostic accuracy by uncovering structures that two dimensional imaging cannot reveal. When evaluating persistent symptoms, CBCT allows the clinician to visualize anatomical complexities such as narrow isthmuses, untreated accessory canals, and apical deltas that harbor residual microorganisms. It also exposes small vertical fractures or subtle bone defects that remain invisible on conventional radiographs. However, CBCT interpretation must remain biologically grounded. An area of postoperative radiolucency that appears static or decreasing over time is often an indicator of normal healing, even if symptoms persist intermittently. Conversely, an enlarging radiolucency accompanied by increasing pain reflects pathological progression. The clinician's task is to merge radiographic findings with biological patterns in order to differentiate between harmless variations in healing and true indicators of disease.

This integration prevents diagnostic errors and ensures that interventions are based on accurate interpretation rather than mechanical reliance on imaging. The clinician who views imaging through a biological lens is better equipped to recognize when symptoms are misleading, when radiographic changes are expected, and when the tissue response is signaling a genuine threat that requires immediate action.

9.2 The Role of Functional Testing in Distinguishing Mechanical and Inflammatory Etiologies

While imaging and symptom history are essential, functional testing often provides the decisive evidence needed to distinguish mechanical irritation from inflammatory or microbial pathology. These tests allow clinicians to observe how the tooth behaves under controlled stimuli, revealing patterns that subjective descriptions cannot fully capture. For example, a tooth that produces sharp pain only during biting indicates stress within the periodontal ligament rather than deep inflammatory pressure from the apical region. This pain pattern points toward occlusal overload, high contact, or structural compromise such as a cracked cusp. When the same tooth produces lingering pain without chewing or biting, the clinician must consider deeper inflammatory involvement.

Bite tests using materials such as cotton rolls, articulating paper, or plastic bite sticks allow precise localization of mechanical sensitivity. Pain triggered only on one cusp suggests a localized structural issue, while pain distributed across the entire biting surface suggests generalized ligament inflammation. Percussion testing offers another layer of insight. Sensitivity to vertical tapping indicates inflammation within the ligament or apical tissues, while horizontal tapping may reveal cracks or structural compromise. Combined testing clarifies whether the source of discomfort is mechanical, inflammatory, or microbial, guiding the clinician toward appropriate treatment pathways.

Thermal testing, although less common after obturation, can still offer valuable diagnostic clues when symptoms persist. For example, a lingering cold response after root canal therapy may signal coronal leakage that reintroduces microorganisms into the canal system. A heat response may indicate pressure buildup within inflamed periapical tissues. These distinctions help clinicians avoid misinterpreting symptoms and ensure that interventions target the true cause of the problem.

Functional testing therefore bridges the gap between clinical suspicion and clinical confirmation. It transforms vague patient descriptions into concrete diagnostic patterns that clinicians can interpret with precision. By incorporating functional testing into every advanced assessment pathway, clinicians strengthen their diagnostic accuracy, reduce unnecessary retreatments, and provide patients with care that is both targeted and evidence based.

CHAPTER 10

Integrated Strategies for Long Term Prevention of Post Obturation Pain and Swelling

L ong term prevention of post obturation pain and swelling depends on the clinician's ability to integrate biological knowledge, diagnostic accuracy, technical precision, and patient centered care into a cohesive framework. Each phase of root canal therapy influences the next, and the quality of decisions made during treatment has a direct impact on the stability of periapical tissues long after obturation is complete. This chapter explores the preventive strategies that form the foundation for sustainable success, emphasizing the importance of meticulous technique, thoughtful material selection, reinforced infection control, and continuous patient monitoring.

Preventive strategies begin with a precise understanding of canal anatomy. The complexity of the root canal system is a major contributor to postoperative complications. Every missed canal, untreated isthmus, or insufficiently instrumented segment creates an environment where microorganisms persist and trigger inflammation. Modern endodontic practice requires the clinician to use magnification, advanced illumination, and comprehensive anatomical knowledge to locate and treat all canals effectively. Proper canal scouting through careful tactile feedback and preoperative radiographic analysis ensures a complete understanding of canal morphology before shaping and cleaning begin. By approaching instrumentation with anatomical precision, the clinician sets the stage for predictable outcomes and minimizes the risk of microbial persistence.

Once anatomical complexities are addressed, disinfection becomes the central preventive strategy. Irrigation is not a secondary step in endodontics but the primary mechanism for destroying microorganisms and removing organic debris. Sodium hypochlorite, when activated with agitation techniques such as ultrasonic activation or negative pressure delivery, penetrates canal irregularities where files cannot reach. Chlorhexidine offers residual antimicrobial activity when used in specific situations, while EDTA facilitates the removal of smear layer that may otherwise shield microorganisms from irrigants. Prevention of postoperative pain and swelling relies on the careful sequencing of irrigants and selection of activation methods that maximize antimicrobial penetration without causing tissue irritation. When irrigation is performed with precision, the microbial load is reduced to a level that significantly lowers the risk of postoperative complications.

Another preventive element involves shaping the canal in a manner that promotes effective irrigation and obturation without causing unnecessary structural damage. Over instrumentation risks debris extrusion into periapical tissues, which can trigger acute inflammation. Under instrumentation allows debris and microorganisms to remain trapped within canal walls. The clinician must strike a balance between enlarging the canal sufficiently for irrigant penetration and preserving the structural integrity of the tooth. This balance is essential for preventing postoperative symptoms and ensuring long term strength of the root.

Obturation itself plays a crucial role in long term prevention. The goal is to create a three dimensional seal within the canal system that blocks microbial ingress and prevents fluid exchange. Gutta percha paired with bioceramic sealers offers excellent sealing ability and biocompatibility, allowing for stable long term outcomes. However, obturation should only be performed when the canal is fully disinfected, dry, and ready to receive filling material. Premature obturation in the presence of inflammation or exudate increases the likelihood of postoperative flare ups. Conversely, delaying obturation in certain cases can expose the canal to contamination. Prevention requires clinical judgment to determine the appropriate timing based on tissue response and clinical findings.

Even the most meticulously executed root canal can fail if coronal integrity is not preserved. Coronal leakage is one of the most preventable causes of postoperative complications. A well sealed restoration is essential for protecting the canal system from salivary bacteria that can infiltrate even small gaps or worn margins. Temporary restorations must be placed carefully and replaced promptly with permanent restorations that demonstrate high marginal integrity. Restorations that permit microleakage undermine the entire endodontic procedure and can lead to reinfection that manifests as pain, swelling, or radiographic changes. Prevention requires the clinician to prioritize coronal protection as an inseparable extension of endodontic therapy.

Infection control protocols also play an important role in preventing postoperative complications. Sterile instrumentation, proper rubber dam isolation, and contamination free irrigant delivery prevent iatrogenic introduction of microorganisms during treatment. When these protocols are executed consistently, the risk of postoperative infection decreases significantly. Prevention is not a single action but a continuous process woven throughout every step of care.

Patient factors must also be considered in long term prevention. Patients with systemic conditions such as diabetes, immune disorders, or vascular impairment experience slower healing and may display heightened inflammatory responses. These patients require tailored treatment plans that include closer monitoring, extended healing timelines, and in some cases, modified pharmacologic support. Effective communication with the patient regarding expectations and healing patterns prevents anxiety, reduces perceived pain intensity, and supports a cooperative approach to postoperative care.

Preventive strategies also extend beyond the treatment itself. Follow up evaluations allow the clinician to monitor healing, identify early signs of complications, and intervene before symptoms escalate. Radiographic reassessment reveals whether periapical tissues are improving, stable, or deteriorating. These evaluations provide valuable feedback for refining clinical technique and improving outcomes for future cases. Prevention is an ongoing commitment that continues long after the obturation is complete.

Ultimately, long term prevention of post obturation pain and swelling relies on the synergy between knowledge, technique, and clinical judgment. The clinician must understand the biological events occurring within the canal and periapical tissues, anticipate challenges associated with anatomical complexity, apply disinfection and obturation techniques with precision, and maintain coronal protection to prevent reinfection. When these strategies are integrated into a unified preventive philosophy, the likelihood of postoperative complications decreases significantly, and the durability of treatment outcomes increases.

10.1 Strengthening the Coronal Seal as a Primary Defense Against Reinfection

The integrity of the coronal seal plays a decisive role in preventing long term postoperative complications. Even when root canal therapy is executed with exceptional precision, the treatment can fail if the coronal barrier allows salivary microorganisms to reenter the canal system. Coronal leakage is often underestimated in clinical practice, yet it remains one of the leading preventable causes of reinfection. Bacteria require only microscopic gaps to infiltrate restorative materials, and once contamination occurs, the microbial load can reestablish itself deep within the obturated canals. This leads to inflammation that may manifest as tenderness, swelling, or radiographic deterioration months after treatment.

A strong coronal seal begins with proper case sequencing and meticulous temporary restoration. Temporary materials should provide adequate strength, resistance to wear, and minimal microleakage. Cotton pellets must be placed judiciously to avoid compressing the material or leaving excessive space that weakens the restoration. Long term temporization should be avoided whenever possible because temporary materials degrade over time and allow bacteria to penetrate. After obturation, prompt placement of a permanent restoration is essential. Composite resins, full coverage crowns, or onlays should be selected based on the remaining tooth structure, functional demands, and esthetic requirements.

Permanent restorations must demonstrate tight marginal adaptation, proper contour, and resistance to breakdown under occlusal forces. Marginal gaps, fractured cusps, or incomplete curing can undermine the coronal seal and compromise treatment longevity. The clinician must also consider advanced restorative strategies such as bonded cores or fiber reinforcement in structurally compromised teeth. By prioritizing the coronal seal at every stage, clinicians create a robust barrier that safeguards the canal system and significantly reduces the likelihood of reinfection and postoperative symptoms.

10.2 Optimizing Irrigation Dynamics to Enhance Microbial Control and Tissue Compatibility

Irrigation is one of the most powerful tools for preventing postoperative complications because it determines the extent of microbial elimination within the canal system. Instrumentation alone cannot reach the complex network of lateral canals, isthmuses, fins, and dendritic spaces where microorganisms reside. Effective prevention relies on irrigation strategies that maximize antimicrobial penetration while minimizing tissue irritation. Sodium hypochlorite remains the gold standard due to its ability to dissolve organic material and destroy microorganisms, but its effectiveness depends on how it is delivered and activated within the canal.

Dynamic irrigation systems enhance the movement of irrigant solutions, allowing them to penetrate areas that files cannot access. Techniques such as ultrasonic activation create acoustic streaming and cavitation that lift debris from canal walls and expose deeper layers of biofilm. Negative pressure irrigation draws the solution into narrow canal spaces while preventing accidental extrusion into periapical tissues. These methods produce a cleaner canal environment and reduce the risk of postoperative flare ups caused by residual microbial products.

Proper sequencing of irrigants further enhances preventive outcomes. Sodium hypochlorite should be followed by EDTA to remove the smear layer and expose dentinal tubules for deeper penetration. In cases where chemical irritation may contribute to postoperative discomfort, clinicians must assess irrigant concentration and exposure time carefully. Higher concentrations offer increased antimicrobial power but may irritate periapical tissues if inadvertently extruded. Balanced irrigation, guided by clinical judgment, ensures that antimicrobial action is maximized without compromising tissue compatibility.

When irrigation dynamics are optimized, the canal environment becomes significantly more resistant to postoperative inflammation. Preventive strategies that emphasize irrigant activation, proper sequencing, and controlled delivery contribute to long term success and reduce the likelihood of persistent pain or swelling.

REVIEWS

1. Dr. Bukola Adeniran, Consultant Endodontist, Ibadan

This book provides one of the clearest explanations of postoperative endodontic complications that I have seen in recent literature. The author blends scientific depth with practical guidance in a way that supports day to day clinical decision making. The chapters on etiology and inflammatory responses are exceptionally well structured and will benefit clinicians who want to improve both outcomes and patient comfort.

2. Dr. Emmanuel Chidera Okonkwo, Lecturer in Restorative Dentistry, University of Nigeria

Many texts focus on technique without addressing the biological events that follow treatment. This book fills that gap with impressive academic strength. The preventive strategies and diagnostic frameworks are explained in a manner that is both evidence based and clinically useful.

3. Dr. Zainab Bello, General Dental Practitioner, Kaduna

In a busy clinical environment, postoperative discomfort can quickly become a source of anxiety for patients. This book has helped me refine how I approach these cases. The management protocols, medication guidance, and stepwise assessment tools are clearly articulated and easy to apply in practice. It has become an essential reference in my clinic.

4. Dr. Tunde Ajambele, Oral and Maxillofacial Surgery Trainee, Lagos

The strength of this book lies in its balanced combination of scientific detail and clinical relevance. The explanations of microbial persistence, apical irritation, and tissue level responses are excellent. These insights have enhanced my understanding of how postoperative symptoms develop and how they can be controlled. It is a significant contribution to dental literature in Nigeria.

5. Dr. Oyinade Afolabi, Endodontic Research Associate, Ilorin

This work stands out as a thoughtful and methodologically sound exploration of postoperative challenges in endodontics. The author presents complex ideas in a clear and structured way, making the book useful for both researchers and clinicians. I found the sections on retreatment and long term outcome evaluation especially valuable. This text deserves recognition for its scholarly merit.

REFERENCES

Arias, A., Azabal, M., Hidalgo, J. J., & de la Macorra, J. C. (2013). Relationship between postendodontic pain, tooth diagnostic factors, and clinical variables. *Journal of Endodontics, 39*(3), 300–304. https://doi.org/10.1016/j.joen.2012.11.008

Bergenholtz, G., Horsted-Bindslev, P., & Reit, C. (Eds.). (2010). *Textbook of endodontology* (2nd ed.). Wiley Blackwell.

Cohen, S., & Hargreaves, K. M. (Eds.). (2011). *Pathways of the pulp* (10th ed.). Mosby Elsevier.

El Mubarak, A. H., Abu-bakr, N. H., & Ibrahim, Y. E. (2010). Postoperative pain in multiple-visit and single-visit root canal treatment. *Journal of Endodontics, 36*(1), 36–39. https://doi.org/10.1016/j.joen.2009.09.041

European Society of Endodontology. (2006). Quality guidelines for endodontic treatment: Consensus report from the European Society of Endodontology. *International Endodontic Journal, 39*(12), 921–930. https://doi.org/10.1111/j.1365-2591.2006.01180.x

Fouad, A. F., & Rivera, E. M. (2019). *Clinical decision-making in endodontics* (2nd ed.). Wiley Blackwell.

Gomes, B. P. F. A., Vianna, M. E., Zaia, A. A., Almeida, J. F. A., Souza-Filho, F. J., & Ferraz, C. C. R. (2015). Endodontic microbiology: Biological considerations and clinical applications. *Brazilian Dental Journal, 26*(1), 1–10. https://doi.org/10.1590/0103-6440201302443

Gutmann, J. L., & Solomon, E. S. (2014). Pain and healing following endodontic therapy: A clinical and biological review. *Endodontic Topics, 30*(1), 73–98. https://doi.org/10.1111/etp.12053

Hargreaves, K. M., Abbott, P. V., & Walton, R. E. (2016). *Seltzer and Bender's dental pulp* (2nd ed.). Quintessence Publishing.

Keiser, K., & Hargreaves, K. M. (2002). Building effective pain management strategies for endodontic patients. *Endodontic Topics, 3*(1), 93–105. https://doi.org/10.1034/j.1601-1546.2002.30108.x

Manfredi, M., Figini, L., Gagliani, M., & Lodi, G. (2016). Single versus multiple visits for endodontic treatment: Systematic review of randomized clinical trials. *European Journal of Dentistry, 10*(1), 58–66. https://doi.org/10.4103/1305-7456.175685

Nair, P. N. R. (2006). On the causes of persistent apical periodontitis: A review. *International Endodontic Journal, 39*(4), 249–281. https://doi.org/10.1111/j.1365-2591.2006.01099.x

Patel, S., Durack, C., Abella, F., Roig, M., Shemesh, H., & Lambrechts, P. (2015). Cone beam computed tomography in endodontics: A review. *International Endodontic Journal, 48*(1), 3–15. https://doi.org/10.1111/iej.12270

Siqueira, J. F., & Rôças, I. N. (2008). Clinical implications and microbiology of bacterial persistence after treatment procedures. *Journal of Endodontics, 34*(11), 1291–1301. https://doi.org/10.1016/j.joen.2008.07.028

Siqueira, J. F., & Rôças, I. N. (2014). *Treatment of endodontic infections*. Quintessence Publishing.

Torabinejad, M., Fouad, A. F., & Walton, R. E. (2019). *Endodontics: Principles and practice* (6th ed.). Elsevier.

Walton, R., & Fouad, A. (1992). Endodontic interappointment flare ups: A prospective study of incidence and related factors. *Journal of Endodontics, 18*(4), 172–177. https://doi.org/10.1016/S0099-2399(06)81413-5

www.ingramcontent.com/pod-product-compliance
Lightning Source LLC
Chambersburg PA
CBHW021539260326
41914CB00001B/77